Current Management Guidelines in Thoracic Surgery

Guest Editor

M. BLAIR MARSHALL, MD

THORACIC SURGERY CLINICS

www.thoracic.theclinics.com

Consulting Editor
MARK K. FERGUSON, MD

February 2012 • Volume 22 • Number 1

SAUNDERS an imprint of ELSEVIER, Inc.

W.B. SAUNDERS COMPANY
A Division of Elsevier Inc.

1600 John F. Kennedy Boulevard • Suite 1800 • Philadelphia, Pennsylvania 19103-2899

http://www.theclinics.com

THORACIC SURGERY CLINICS Volume 22, Number 1
February 2012 ISSN 1547-4127, ISBN-13: 978-1-4557-3943-1

Editor: Barbara Cohen-Kligerman

Thoracic Surgery Clinics (ISSN 1547-4127) is published quarterly by Elsevier Inc., 360 Park Avenue South, New York, NY 10010-1710. Months of publication are February, May, August, and November. Business and editorial offices: 1600 John F. Kennedy Boulevard, Suite 1800, Philadelphia, PA 19103-2899. Periodicals postage paid at New York, NY, and additional mailing offices. Subscription prices are $322.00 per year (US individuals), $416.00 per year (US institutions), $154.00 per year (US Students), $400.00 per year (Canadian individuals), $526.00 per year (Canadian institutions), $209.00 per year (Canadian and foreign students), $426.00 per year (foreign individuals), and $526.00 per year (foreign institutions). Foreign air speed delivery is included in all Clinics' subscription prices. All prices are subject to change without notice. **POSTMASTER:** Send address changes to Thoracic Surgery Clinics, Elsevier Health Sciences Division, Subscription Customer Service, 3251 Riverport Lane, Maryland Heights, MO 63043. **Customer Service (orders, claims, online, change of address): Telephone: 1-800-654-2452 (U.S. and Canada); 314-447-8871 (outside U.S. and Canada). Fax: 314-447-8029. Email: journalscustomerservice-usa@elsevier.com (for print support); journalsonlinesupport-usa@elsevier.com (for online support).**

Reprints. For copies of 100 or more, of articles in this publication, please contact Commercial Rights Department, Elsevier Inc., 360 Park Avenue South, New York, NY 10010-1710. Tel: (212) 633-3812; Fax: (212) 462-1935; E-mail: reprints@elsevier.com.

Thoracic Surgery Clinics is covered in *MEDLINE/PubMed (Index Medicus)* and *EMBASE/Excerpta Medica*.

Printed and bound by CPI Group (UK) Ltd, Croydon, CR0 4YY

Transferred to Digital Print 2012

Contributors

CONSULTING EDITOR

MARK K. FERGUSON, MD
Professor of Surgery, Section of Cardiac and
Thoracic Surgery, The University of Chicago
Medical Center, Chicago, Illinois

GUEST EDITOR

M. BLAIR MARSHALL, MD
Associate Professor of Surgery, Georgetown
University School of Medicine; Chief, Division
of Thoracic Surgery, Department of Surgery,
Georgetown University Medical Center,
Washington, DC

AUTHORS

JUSTIN D. BLASBERG, MD
Department of Cardiothoracic Surgery,
Massachusetts General Hospital, Boston,
Massachusetts

ALESSANDRO BRUNELLI, MD
Chair, Section Minimally Invasive Thoracic
Surgery, Division of Thoracic Surgery, Ospedali
Riuniti Ancona, Ancona, Italy

AYESHA S. BRYANT, MSPH, MD
Assistant Professor, Division of Cardiothoracic
Surgery, Department of Surgery, University of
Alabama at Birmingham, Birmingham,
Alabama

ROBERT J. CERFOLIO, MD, FACS, FCCP
Professor of Surgery, Chief of Section of
Thoracic Surgery, JH Estes Chair for Lung
Cancer Research, Division of Cardiothoracic
Surgery, University of Alabama at Birmingham,
Birmingham, Alabama

STEPHANIE H. CHANG, MD
General Surgery Resident, Division of
Cardiothoracic Surgery, Washington University
in St Louis School of Medicine, St Louis,
Missouri

PAUL M. CLAIBORNE
The University of Texas Medical School at
Houston, Houston, Texas

ELIZABETH A. DAVID, MD
Cardiothoracic Surgery Resident, University of
Texas MD Anderson Cancer Center, Houston,
Texas

MALCOLM M. DECAMP, MD
Fowler McCormick Professor of Surgery,
Division of Thoracic Surgery, Northwestern
Memorial Hospital, Northwestern University
Feinberg School of Medicine, Chicago, Illinois

ALBERTO DE HOYOS, MD
Assistant Professor of Surgery, Division of
Thoracic Surgery, Northwestern Memorial
Hospital, Northwestern University Feinberg
School of Medicine, Chicago, Illinois

JESSICA S. DONINGTON, MD
Director of Thoracic Surgery, Bellevue
Hospital; Assistant Professor, Department of
Cardiothoracic Surgery, NYU School of
Medicine, New York, New York

HIRAN C. FERNANDO, MD, FRCS
Department of Cardiothoracic Surgery, Boston University School of Medicine, Boston, Massachusetts

CLARA S. FOWLER, MSLS
Manager, Information Services, Research Medical Library, The University of Texas MD Anderson Cancer Center, Houston, Texas

JOHN R. GOLDBLUM, MD
Professor of Pathology, Cleveland Clinic Lerner College of Medicine; Chairman, Department of Anatomic Pathology, Cleveland Clinic, Cleveland, Ohio

ALEXANDER S. KRUPNICK, MD
Assistant Professor of Surgery, Division of Cardiothoracic Surgery, Washington University in St Louis School of Medicine, St Louis, Missouri

JOHN C. KUCHARCZUK, MD
Associate Professor of Surgery, Division of Thoracic Surgery, Hospital of the University of Pennsylvania, Philadelphia, Pennsylvania

M. BLAIR MARSHALL, MD
Associate Professor of Surgery, Georgetown University School of Medicine; Chief, Division of Thoracic Surgery, Department of Surgery, Georgetown University Medical Center, Washington, DC

MARISSA M. MONTGOMERY, BA
Boston University School of Medicine, Boston, Massachusetts

AVEDIS MENESHIAN, MD
Assistant Professor of Surgery and Oncology, Division of Thoracic Surgery, The Johns Hopkins Medical Institutions, Baltimore, Maryland

ROBERT E. MERRITT, MD
Assistant Professor of Cardiothoracic Surgery, Division of Thoracic Surgery, Department of Cardiothoracic Surgery, Stanford University School of Medicine, Stanford, California

ALESSANDRO MORABITO, MD
Lung Cancer Multidisciplinary Team, Division of Medical Oncology, Department of Thoracic Surgery and Oncology, National Cancer Institute, Pascale Foundation, Naples, Italy

PAOLO MUTO, MD
Lung Cancer Multidisciplinary Team, Division of Radiation Oncology, National Cancer Institute, Pascale Foundation, Naples, Italy

CHAITAN K. NARSULE, MD
Department of Cardiothoracic Surgery, Boston University School of Medicine, Boston, Massachusetts

FRANCIS C. NICHOLS, MD
Chair, Division of General Thoracic Surgery; Consultant, Division of General Thoracic Surgery; Associate Professor of Surgery, Mayo Clinic, Rochester, Minnesota

THOMAS W. RICE, MD
Professor of Surgery, Cleveland Clinic Lerner College of Medicine; The Daniel and Karen Lee Endowed Chair in Thoracic Surgery, Department of Thoracic and Cardiovascular Surgery, Cleveland Clinic, Cleveland, Ohio

GAETANO ROCCO, MD, FRCSEd
Lung Cancer Multidisciplinary Team, Division of Thoracic Surgery, Department of Thoracic Surgery and Oncology, National Cancer Institute, Pascale Foundation, Naples, Italy

JOSEPH B. SHRAGER, MD
Professor of Cardiothoracic Surgery, Chief of the Division of Thoracic Surgery, Department of Cardiothoracic Surgery, Stanford University School of Medicine, Stanford; Division of Thoracic Surgery, VA Palo Alto Health Care System, Palo Alto, California

CAROL SOUTHARD, RN, MSN
Northwestern Integrative Medicine, Northwestern Memorial Physicians Group, Chicago, Illinois

ARA A. VAPORCIYAN, MD, FACS
Professor and Deputy Chair, Director of Clinical Education and Training, Department of Thoracic and Cardiovascular Surgery, University of Texas MD Anderson Cancer Center, Houston, Texas

STEPHEN C. YANG, MD, FACS, FCCP
The Arthur B. and Patricia B. Modell Professor of Thoracic Surgery; Professor and Chief of Thoracic Surgery, The Johns Hopkins Medical Institutions, Baltimore, Maryland

Contents

Preface: Current Management Guidelines in Thoracic Surgery xi

M. Blair Marshall

Perioperative Smoking Cessation 1

Alberto de Hoyos, Carol Southard, and Malcolm M. DeCamp

Smoking is the leading cause of preventable death worldwide. Smoking cessation programs that include counseling and pharmacotherapy have been proved to be effective in achieving long-standing abstinence. Smoking cessation is associated with significant improvements in quality of life, mortality, life expectancy, and postsurgical complication rates. Contrary to general belief, smoking cessation close to the time of elective surgery does not increase the risk of pulmonary complications. Longer-term quit rates are generally higher in cohorts who quit in anticipation of surgery compared with those quitting for general health considerations. A team approach and adherence to the guidelines for smoking cessation improves long-term chances of success.

Prophylaxis and Management of Atrial Fibrillation After General Thoracic Surgery 13

Robert E. Merritt and Joseph B. Shrager

Atrial fibrillation (AF) commonly affects patients after general thoracic surgery. Postoperative AF increases hospital stay and charges. Effective prophylaxis and treatment is the goal. Calcium channel blockers prevent postoperative AF. Beta blockers are a less viable choice. Amiodarone prophylaxis should be avoided in patients with pulmonary dysfunction or who require pneumonectomy. In management of AF, a brief trial of rate-control agents is appropriate; however, chemical cardioversion with rhythm-control agents should be instituted after 24 hours. High-risk patients with history of stroke or transient ischemic attack, or with two or more risk factors for thromboembolism should receive anticoagulation therapy.

Deep Vein Thrombosis/Pulmonary Embolism: Prophylaxis, Diagnosis, and Management 25

Alessandro Brunelli

Thoracic surgery patients should be regarded at high risk for postoperative venous thromboembolism (VTE). VTE mechanical and pharmacologic prophylaxis with low molecular weight heparin, or low-dose unfractionated heparin or fondaparinux (Arixtra) is therefore strongly recommended. Pharmacologic prophylaxis should be extended to 4 weeks after major cancer surgery. Pulmonary embolism should be always managed with anticoagulation, in addition to thrombolytic therapy, in patients presenting with cardiogenic shock or persistent arterial hypotension.

The Management of Anticoagulants Perioperatively 29

Robert J. Cerfolio and Ayesha S. Bryant

Perioperative management of anticoagulants requires one to balance the patient's risk factors for operative bleeding, the type of operation to be performed, and the patient's risk of thromboembolism. At present, no set algorithm exists for the perioperative management of all the anticoagulants. In this article, we address the perioperative management of the most commonly used anticoagulants seen in practice today, such as warfarin, heparin, dabigatran, clopidogrel, and aspirin, for the most commonly performed general thoracic operations.

Perioperative Antibiotics in Thoracic Surgery

35

Stephanie H. Chang and Alexander S. Krupnick

No official guidelines exist for perioperative antibiotic use in noncardiac thoracic surgery. Despite some conflicting data and few randomized clinical trials there exists strong evidence supporting the use of perioperative antibiotic prophylaxis in pulmonary resection. This article discusses the evidence-based indications for antibiotic prophylaxis after lung resection, esophageal surgery, and lung transplantation.

Physiologic Evaluation of Lung Resection Candidates

47

Elizabeth A. David and M. Blair Marshall

This article reviews an evidence-based approach to the physiologic evaluation of patients under consideration for surgical resection of lung cancer. Adequate physiologic evaluation often includes a multidisciplinary evaluation, with complete identification of risk factors for perioperative complications and long-term disability including cardiovascular risk, assessment of pulmonary function, and smoking cessation counseling. Consideration of tumor-related anatomic obstruction, atelectasis, or vascular occlusion may alter measurements. Careful preoperative physiologic assessment helps to identify patients at increased risk of morbidity and mortality after lung resection. These evaluations are helpful in identifying patients who may not benefit from surgical management of their lung cancer.

Management of Early Stage Non–Small Cell Lung Cancer in High-Risk Patients

55

Jessica S. Donington and Justin D. Blasberg

The preferred treatment of stage I non–small cell lung cancer (NSCLC) is anatomic resection with systematic mediastinal lymph node evaluation. However, 20% of patients with operable lung cancer are not candidates for this type of resection. Recent advancements in radiology-guided technologies have expanded the treatment options for high-risk patients with early-stage NSCLC. There has simultaneously been resurgence in interest and refinement of indications and techniques for sublobar resection in this population. While these treatments appear to have decreased peri-procedural morbidity and mortality, their oncologic efficacy compared to that of lobectomy remains to be determined.

Induction Therapy for Lung Cancer: Sailing Across the Pillars of Hercules

67

Gaetano Rocco, Alessandro Morabito, and Paolo Muto

In spite of numerous clinical trials, the jury is still out on the value of induction therapy for locally advanced lung cancer. We elected to address this topic from the multifaceted views of the clinicians often involved in lung cancer management and according the most recent views on locally advanced NSCLC. The concept of a prognostic stratification of N2 disease subsets, especially single vs multiple zone, has been introduced and this may lead to a new interpretation of locally advanced NSCLC. Ten crucial issues were identified that may have an impact on the approach to patients with locally advanced lung cancer in everyday practice.

Chest Wall Sarcomas and Induction Therapy   77

John C. Kucharczuk

> Chest wall sarcomas are uncommon tumors. The best patient outcomes likely result from a formalized multidisciplinary treatment plan in a specialized center. No clear guidelines exist to determine whether patients with chest wall sarcomas benefit from preoperative adjuvant therapy. Most decisions are made on a case-by-case basis with little available evidence. It is unclear whether established guidelines for the more commonly occurring extremity sarcomas can be appropriately extrapolated to the care of patients with chest wall disease. The single most important factor in local control and long-term survival is a wide, complete, R0 resection.

Induction Therapy for Thymic Malignancies   83

Avedis Meneshian and Stephen C. Yang

> Thymic malignancies are rare tumors of the chest that express a broad range of biological behaviors. Surgery remains the mainstay of therapy, and complete surgical resection is the primary predictor of long-term survival. Although there is a paucity of clinical trials assessing the role of induction/adjuvant chemotherapy and/or radiation therapy in the treatment of thymic malignancies, existing data suggest that induction therapy should be offered for the treatment of advanced-stage disease, and postoperative radiation for specific stages.

Pulmonary Metastasectomy   91

Francis C. Nichols

> The most common cause of cancer death is the development of metastatic disease. Thirty percent of patients eventually develop pulmonary metastases. Randomized control data supporting the commonly accepted practice of surgical pulmonary metastasectomy are lacking. This article focuses on the current surgical management of pulmonary metastases providing the reader with reasonable guidance from the vast literature that exists.

Management of Barrett Esophagus with High-grade Dysplasia   101

Thomas W. Rice and John R. Goldblum

> High-grade dysplasia in Barrett esophagus is a marker for future development of cancer and for the existence of synchronous cancer. A significant problem in management is intraobserver and interobserver variation in the diagnosis of high-grade dysplasia in Barrett esophagus, the natural history of which is poorly understood; thus, treatment decisions are problematic. The ability to preserve the esophagus with endoscopic mucosal ablation or resection and reduce morbidity of treatment has made endoscopic treatment the mainstay of therapy. Esophagectomy is reserved for treatment failures and for high-grade dysplasia not amenable to less aggressive therapies. This article outlines the data supporting current management strategies.

Evidence-Based Review of the Management of Cancers of the Gastroesophageal Junction   109

Chaitan K. Narsule, Marissa M. Montgomery, and Hiran C. Fernando

> The management of localized esophageal cancer has traditionally been surgical resection; yet, despite improvements in outcomes and techniques, survival for patients with esophageal cancer, especially those with evidence of nodal involvement,

remains poor. In this article, we have used an evidence-based approach to define optimal therapy based on clinical stage for esophageal cancer. We review the currently available evidence supporting the use of neoadjuvant and adjuvant therapies for locally advanced esophageal cancer. Additionally, we review the evidence supporting the role of endoscopic therapies, rather than resection, for early-stage esophageal cancer.

Follow-up of Patients with Resected Thoracic Malignancies   **123**

Paul M. Claiborne, Clara S. Fowler, and Ara A. Vaporciyan

The authors have systematically performed a literature search using 8 databases identifying established guidelines for follow-up after resected thoracic malignancies. Seven different societies' (found to have published recommendations for non-small cell lung cancer, esophageal cancer, thymoma, or mesothelioma) guidelines are reviewed in this article. High-quality evidence leading to consistent, strong recommendations among societies has not been found. With the subsequent advancements in surgical treatment and other curative modalities, the ability to detect and intervene with curative therapy at earlier stages of disease in a growing portion of the current patient population will benefit from higher-quality evidence.

Index   **133**

Thoracic Surgery Clinics

FORTHCOMING ISSUES

May 2012

The Lymphatic System in Thoracic Oncology
Federico Venuta, MD, and
Erino A. Rendina, MD, *Guest Editors*

August 2012

Surgical Management of Infectious Pleuropulmonary Diseases
Gaetano Rocco, MD, *Guest Editor*

November 2012

Patient Perspectives in Pulmonary Surgery
Alessandro Brunelli, MD, *Guest Editor*

RECENT ISSUES

November 2011

Advances in the Management of Benign Esophageal Diseases
Blair A. Jobe, MD, *Guest Editor*

August 2011

From Residency to Retirement: Building a Successful Thoracic Surgery Career
Sean Grondin, MD, and F.G. Pearson, MD,
Guest Editors

May 2011

Thoracic Anatomy, Part II: Pleura, Mediastinum, Diaphragm, Esophagus
Jean Deslauriers, MD, *Guest Editor*

RELATED INTEREST

Surgical Clinics of North America Volume 20, Issue 4 (October 2011)
Lung Cancer
Mark J. Krasna, MD, *Guest Editor*

Clinics in Chest Medicine Volume 32, Issue 2 (June 2011)
Lung Transplantation
Robert M. Kotloff, MD, *Guest Editor*

READ THE CLINICS ONLINE!

Access your subscription at:
www.theclinics.com

Preface
Current Management Guidelines in Thoracic Surgery

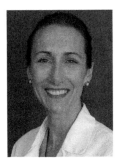

M. Blair Marshall, MD
Guest Editor

Thoracic surgery, as a specialty, covers a great breadth of pathology and care. Thoracic surgeons deal with a variety of conditions affecting multiple organs and systems, from benign processes such as hyperhydrosis and achalasia to multiple malignancies, both primary and metastatic. The optimal management of such a diverse group of patients is very complex. For clinical questions, guidelines have been developed. Guidelines may represent an institutional approach from extensive experience or collaborative efforts within or between societies. They usually serve to provide clarity in an area where multiple strategies may exist or where treatment strategies are evolving. For these guidelines, an exhaustive search of the literature is performed with the level of evidence weighted and statements made about the management of a disease or process based on the best available evidence. The guidelines are vetted and published and serve to set standards and guide care.

THE BEST AVAILABLE EVIDENCE

In a perfect world, every study would be a prospective randomized trial sufficiently powered to demonstrate the advantages or disadvantages of one option over another. In science, answering these types of questions is fairly simple. One uses a clonal population of cells or a colony of identical mice and chooses to alter one variable or another, analyzing the result. Even in these highly controlled settings,

not all treatment groups behave the same. Proliferation or apoptosis rates vary among cell cultures. Some tumors grow on one mouse while the same tumor on a genetically identical mouse might not; yet from what we can tell, the conditions are identical. Results curiously are rarely uniform. We do not know why results vary, other than there are things that we have yet to understand. In the meantime, we average the results and look for statistical significance.

In the practice of medicine, we try to do the same but are forced to work with less uniform conditions. We stratify patients according to disease, stage, or other comparable factors. We accommodate for known variables such as gender, age, comorbidities, etc; however, many variables that we have yet to understand go unaccounted for. We know that the best protocol is a prospective randomized one, but in the establishment of many guidelines, these are few and far between.

This is particularly challenging when the disease process is rare, as we are unable to treat coherently either a uniform population or a population uniformly. In the management of many patients and their pathology, we continue to have so many unanswered questions. At times, the morbidity or mortality associated with a disease is such that aggressive treatments are added on top of the "standard of care," looking for the next therapeutic breakthrough. In these situations, we maximize support for patients who are being

Thorac Surg Clin 22 (2012) xi–xii
doi:10.1016/j.thorsurg.2011.10.001

thoracic.theclinics.com

treated in the hope of adding even more treatments, striving to make an impact in the natural history of the disease.

In other settings, such as high-grade dysplasia, where the previous standard was associated with significant morbidity and long-term effects, we strive to minimize physiologic impact and obtain equivalent oncologic outcomes. All along we recognize that we are unable to predict the future. Until time tells, we will not know if the correct decision was made.

Over the past several years, we have been able to increase our understanding of additional differences between patients and their disease processes. We now have microarrays, genetic markers, and mutations as well as the knowledge of additional variables previously unidentified or unrecognized. Going forward, we stand to gain so much knowledge at such a fast rate given the advances in technology and science. In the midst of all this, we look to guidelines to help us to optimize the management of our patients. Guidelines, though, are just that, guidelines. They provide us with the scientific foundation on which to treat our patients. We as surgeons continue to practice the art of medicine, which is how guidelines, developed from a variety of studies on an impurely uniform patient population, should apply to our individual patient. It is here that we have asked each of the authors to provide their insight on the use of guidelines and the optimal management of our patients within the context of their expertise.

This issue represents significant efforts of others, especially the authors. I would sincerely like to thank all of the authors for their tireless efforts in the production of this edition. I greatly appreciate their efforts. I am indebted to the staff at Elsevier, in particular, Barbara Cohen-Kligerman and Ruth Malwitz, for their organization and follow-up skills, as without these, the issue would not have been possible. Last, I am so very grateful to Consulting Editor, Dr Mark Ferguson, for giving me the opportunity to act as Guest Editor and for all of his guidance and assistance in the development of this issue.

M. Blair Marshall, MD
Division of Thoracic Surgery
Department of Surgery
Georgetown University Medical Center
4 PHC, 3800 Reservoir Road, NW
Washington, DC 20007, USA

E-mail address:
Mbm5@gunet.georgetown.edu

Perioperative Smoking Cessation

Alberto de Hoyos, MD[a], Carol Southard, RN, MSN[b],
Malcolm M. DeCamp, MD[a],*

KEYWORDS

- Smoking cessation • Pharmacotherapy • Counseling
- Preoperative

It is impossible to overstate the impact of tobacco use on national and global health, because tobacco consumption remains the largest single preventable cause of death in the world. Worldwide, tobacco causes approximately 1 in 10 deaths, and by 2030 this figure is expected to rise to 1 in 6, or 10 million deaths each year.[1,2] Globally, smoking is still a very common practice, with 48% of the world's men and 10% of women classified as habitual smokers.[3] The prevalence of smoking in the United States has declined among men from 57% to 23% and among women from 34% to 18% during the period between 1955 and 2005.[4] Although cigarette consumption has declined in recent years, an estimated 21% of United States adults smoked in 2004.[5] The highest rate of decline in smoking occurred between 1965 and 1990 and seemed to be related to public health measures, such as bans on smoking in public places, increased cigarette taxes, mass media antismoking campaigns, and restrictions on marketing of cigarettes. Since 1990, however, there seems to be minimal progress, indicating a need for new strategies as the number of smokers in the United States remains greater than 43 million.

The economic and healthcare costs of tobacco use in the United Stated exceed $400 billion annually.[6] Smoking cessation is one of the most effective ways to promote public health and reduce healthcare costs.[7] The 2008 report from the surgeon general concluded that tobacco-dependence treatments are effective across a broad range of populations and recommended that pharmacotherapy be offered to all cigarette smokers. Despite substantiation that evidence-based effective interventions exist and that most adult smokers want to quit, only a small proportion of tobacco users are offered assistance or receive treatment. This disconnect epitomizes a significant quality of healthcare predicament.

Of the approximately 6 billion people alive today, half a billion people will be killed by tobacco products. By 2020, tobacco is expected to kill more people than any single disease.[8,9] Half of these deaths will occur in people in their middle age, depriving societies of their most productive workers and burdening healthcare systems. The World Health Organization Framework Convention on Tobacco Control aims to reduce the health consequences of tobacco use through the worldwide implementation of evidence-based tobacco control actions.[10] The Framework Convention on Tobacco Control treaty is the first global plan attempting to regulate the tobacco industry, and it has now been signed by 168 countries, making it the most widely accepted treaty in United Nations history.

Smoking causes more than 435,000 premature deaths in the United States alone.[11] It is estimated that smoking eventually kills one in two smokers and that the sequelae of tobacco dependence kill approximately 10% of adults worldwide. No other product exists that causes the premature death of 50% of those who use it as intended.[12] Current smokers have nearly three times the risk

a Division of Thoracic Surgery, Northwestern Memorial Hospital, Northwestern University Feinberg School of Medicine, 676 North Saint Clair Street, Suite 650, Chicago, IL 60611, USA
b Northwestern Integrative Medicine, Northwestern Memorial Physicians Group, Chicago, IL, USA
* Corresponding author. 676 North Saint Clair Street, Suite 650, Chicago, IL 60611.
E-mail address: mdecamp@nmh.org

Thorac Surg Clin 22 (2012) 1–12
doi:10.1016/j.thorsurg.2011.09.006

of premature death compared with nonsmokers. Smokers also have up to a 20-fold increase in the risk of developing lung cancer compared with lifetime nonsmokers.[13] In addition, smoking accounts for at least 23.9% of all cancer deaths (33.4% men and 9.6% women) including carcinoma of the lung, lip, oral cavity, pharynx, larynx, esophagus, pancreas, uterine cervix, kidney, bladder, and stomach.[14,15] On average, male smokers lose 13.2 years of life expectancy, and female smokers lose 14.5 years.

SMOKING CESSATION
Benefits of Quitting

The positive effects of smoking cessation are measurable almost immediately. As soon as 20 minutes after the last cigarette, blood pressure decreases and peripheral vasoconstriction is reduced. After 8 hours, carbon monoxide levels drop to normal. After 24 hours the chance of a coronary artery occlusive event is reduced. After 1 to 9 months, respiratory ciliary function returns to normal allowing for appropriate clearance of mucus and particulate matter. In addition, patients with lung cancer who quit also experience decreased fatigue and shortness of breath and improved performance status, appetite, sleep, and mood.[16] The risk of coronary heart disease drops to half of that of a smoker after 1 year of abstinence and to the level of a nonsmoker after 15 years. The risk of stroke is reduced to the level of a nonsmoker after 5 to 15 years of abstinence.[17] Perhaps most significant is a sharp reduction in mortality because on average, smokers die 13 to 14 years earlier than nonsmokers. Other benefits of quitting include reduction in all-cause mortality,[18] improved response to chemotherapy and radiation,[19,20] improved quality of life,[21] reduction in second primary lung cancer,[22] and decreased postoperative complications.[23–26]

Smoking Cessation and the Diagnosis of Lung Cancer

At diagnosis of lung cancer, up to 18% of patients are never smokers, 58% are former smokers, and 24% to 40% are current smokers. It is estimated that 20% of patients smoke at the time of lung cancer surgery and about half of these continue to smoke afterward.[27] Despite encouragement to quit smoking and strong intentions to quit, continued tobacco use after diagnosis of lung cancer remains a problem in this population, with an estimated 10% to 20% of patients smoking at some point after diagnosis.[28] Lung cancer surgery may be viewed as a "teachable moment" and cessation programs at the time of surgery have

been shown to be more effective than cohorts attempting to quit for general health benefits.[29]

Quitting Before Surgery

Preoperative smoking cessation seems to offer important benefits in reducing complications. Patients with resected stage I to III non–small cell lung carcinoma who quit smoking after the diagnosis and before the operation have a lower risk of dying compared with smokers who continue to smoke at the time of the operation, suggesting that smoking cessation is beneficial for patients with lung cancer at any time before surgery.[30] A prospective study in general surgery patients demonstrated a predictive role of tobacco smoking on operative mortality, total postoperative complications, admission to the intensive care unit, and lower respiratory tract infections.[23] It is generally believed that 4 to 8 weeks of abstinence from smoking are required to reverse the smoking-induced abnormalities in respiratory cell function. Data from a few observational studies seem to support this concept, noting that 4 to 8 weeks of smoking abstinence before surgery were required to significantly reduce the risk of postoperative pulmonary complications. Indeed, two small studies noted a paradoxic increase in the rate of pulmonary complications among patients who quit or reduced their smoking within 4 to 8 weeks before surgery.[31,32] Recent quitters had a numerically higher but not statistically significant rate of pulmonary morbidity than current smokers, with a relative risk up to 6.7 for smokers who quit smoking within 4 to 8 weeks of surgery. Patients who quit smoking closest to the date of the surgery had the highest rate of pulmonary complications.[33] These data have made it difficult for physicians when counseling patients preoperatively about smoking cessation, when surgery cannot be delayed for an optimal time to allow prolonged smoking cessation.

More recent studies, however, have failed to reproduce the paradoxic increase in pulmonary complications suggesting that it is safe to encourage smoking cessation, regardless of the time, before surgery.[34] In addition, longer periods of smoking cessation seem to be more effective in reducing the incidence or risk of postoperative complications without an increased risk in perioperative complications from short-term cessation.[35] A recent randomized trial demonstrated that on an intention-to-treat analysis the overall complication rate in the control group (smokers) was 41% and in the intervention group (quitters) was 21%, a statistically significant difference favoring the cessation group.[36] A systematic review of randomized clinical trials containing 1194 patients undergoing a variety of surgical procedures demonstrated that intensive preoperative smoking cessation interventions reduced the occurrence of postoperative complications.[24] Despite the conflicting data on the timing of smoking cessation and perioperative pulmonary complications, there is no evidence of increased mortality for recent quitters. A prospective study of 300 patients showed an increased postoperative complication rate in smokers compared with nonsmokers but failed to show any evidence of an increased complication rate in those patient who quit smoking less than 2 months before surgery.[37] There has been a recent emerging body of evidence showing the benefit of preoperative and long-term postoperative smoking cessation.[24,38]

Clinical trials have evaluated smoking cessation interventions at varying times before surgery and found clinically meaningful reductions in complications. A meta-analysis of 6 randomized trials and 15 observational studies demonstrated a relative risk reduction of 41% of postoperative complications. In addition, it was demonstrated that each week of cessation increases the magnitude of effect by 19%.[25] Another recent meta-analysis involving 9 studies and 448 patients also demonstrated that the notion that recent smoking cessation increases the risk of postoperative complications is unfounded and emphasized that physicians should advise their patients to quit at any time before surgery.[26] Risk of hospital death and pulmonary complications after lung cancer resection were increased by smoking and mitigated slowly by perioperative cessation. No optimal interval of smoking cessation was identifiable.[39] The consistent decrease noted in postoperative pulmonary complications as interval of smoking cessation increased suggests that clinicians can safely counsel patients about the benefits of smoking cessation preoperatively, regardless of the interval. Although the relative risk for active smokers or recent quitters is substantial, unduly delaying the operation does not seem justified because of the low overall risk of pulmonary complications and the long-term period during which risk remains elevated. A recent Cochrane review on interventions for preoperative smoking cessation concluded that all smokers should be advised to quit and offered effective interventions, including behavioral support and pharmacotherapy.[40] Contrary to the notion that a short period of smoking cessation results in reduced surgical risk, data demonstrate that even after a year of smoking cessation, risk-adjusted mortality remains elevated compared with lifetime nonsmokers,

suggesting that adverse effects never completely disappear.

CESSATION INTERVENTIONS
Counseling

Techniques for assisting smokers to quit include behavioral counseling to enhance motivation, cognitive therapy to impart adjustment skills, and pharmacologic interventions to reduce nicotine reinforcement or chemically mediated effects of nicotine withdrawal. Although the goal of any intervention is permanent tobacco abstinence, it is rarely achieved with a single treatment. Indeed, relapse is the most likely outcome from any single quit attempt. Most patients do not reach 6 months of abstinence without relapsing and half of those abstinent at 6 months relapse during the subsequent 8 years.[41] Healthcare providers need to be aware that most patients require six or more quit attempts before achieving permanent abstinence and should not view prior attempts as total failures.

Smoking cessation treatment should be conceptualized using a chronic illness model.[42,43] Smoking can be effectively addressed within a busy clinical practice using strategies similar to those used to manage other chronic medical conditions, such as hypertension and diabetes. Medication adjustments and behavioral support should be provided until acceptable therapeutic targets are met and, just as a healthcare provider would not consider discontinuing antidiabetic agents for a patient whose hemoglobin A_{1c} was not at goal, the healthcare professional should not discontinue treatment for tobacco users until permanent quitting is achieved.

The most universally accepted paradigm for treatment of tobacco use and dependence is the Five A's model of the United States Public Health Services (USPHS) Clinical Practice Guideline for Treating Tobacco Use and Dependence (ask, advise, assess, assist, and arrange) (**Table 1**).[44,45] The first step is to identify and document tobacco use status for every patient at every visit. This entails systematically screening all patients for tobacco use (ask). The second step is to stalwartly recommend in a strong and personalized manner to every tobacco user to quit smoking (advise). The third step is to determine willingness to make a quit effort (assess). The fourth step addresses smokers willing to make a quit attempt. These patients should be offered medication and counseling or referral for additional treatment (assist). Finally, the fifth step refers to the necessity for follow-up assistance, either in person or by telephone, beginning the first week after the quit date (arrange).

Table 1
The five As model for treating tobacco use and dependence

Ask about tobacco use	Identify and document tobacco use status for every patient at every visit
Advise to quit	In a clear, strong, and personalized manner urge every tobacco user to quit at every visit
Assess willingness to quit	Determine willingness to make a quit attempt
Assist in quit attempt	Offer medication and provide or refer for counseling or additional treatment to help the patient quit
Arrange follow-up	Arrange for follow-up contacts, beginning the first week after the quit date

Adapted from The Clinical Practice Guideline Treating Tobacco Use and Dependence 2008 Update Panel, Liaisons, and Staff. A clinical practice guideline for treating tobacco use and dependence: 2008 update. A US Public Health Service report. Am J Prev Med 2008;35(2):158–76; with permission.

The updated USPHS Clinical Practice Guideline for Treating Tobacco Use and Dependence[44] endorses a condensed user-friendly model for the healthcare provider who does not have the time, inclination, or expertise to provide the more comprehensive tobacco cessation counseling as recommended by the Five A's guideline. Ask-advise-refer is designed to promote cessation intervention by even the busiest of providers **(Table 2)**.[46] The ask-advise-refer approach integrates the Five A's into an abbreviated intervention that remains consistent with recommended guidelines and is designed such that any healthcare provider can easily integrate meaningful cessation intervention into practice on a routine basis.

Telephone quitlines are a primary resource to further assist patients with the quitting process. These services provide one-on-one counseling, self-help kits, and individualized cessation information at no charge to the patient. Studies have shown that patients who receive quitline counseling are twice as likely to quit compared with patients who quit on their own.[47]

Table 2
The AAR (ask-advise-refer) abbreviated method for tobacco dependence treatment

Tobacco Cessation Counseling	Comment
Ask: Ask if the patient smokes or uses smokeless tobacco products	• Many smokers want to quit and appreciate the encouragement of health professionals
Advise: Advise the patient to quit The benefits of quitting include • Decreased risk of a heart attack, stroke, coronary heart disease; lung, oral, and pharyngeal cancer • Improved sense of taste and smell • Improved circulation and lung function • Improved health of family members	• Smokers are more likely to quit if advised to do so by health professionals • The perioperative examination provides the perfect opportunity to discuss smoking cessation with the patient • Tobacco use is a risk factor for coronary heart disease, heart attack, and lung cancer; second-hand smoke is unhealthy for family members
Refer: Tell the patient that help is a free telephone call away; provide patient with quitline numbers	• Evidence suggests quitline use can more than triple success in quitting • Quitlines provide an easy, fast, and effective way to help smokers quit • By simply identifying smokers, advising them to quit, and sending them to a free telephone service, clinicians can save thousands of lives

Adapted from Zillich AJ, Corelli RL, Hudmon KS. Smoking cessation for the busy clinician. The Rx Consultant 2007;16(8): 1–8; with permission.

Pharmacotherapy

Since 1988, when the US Surgeon General concluded that nicotine is the prime component instigating tobacco addiction, it has also been recognized as the most highly addictive of all chemical substances commonly abused. A chief impediment for most smokers who try to quit is the neurobiology of tobacco dependence, which is fed by the most efficient delivery device of nicotine that exists: the cigarette. Cigarette smoking delivers high concentrations of nicotine to the central nervous system within seconds of each puff. The primary target for nicotine in the central nervous system is the *cx4β2* nicotinic acetylcholine receptor, which when activated by nicotine binding results in the release of dopamine and provides the positive reinforcement observed with cigarette smoking. Smoking one cigarette results in a high level of occupancy of the *cx4β2* nicotinic acetylcholine receptors; three cigarettes completely saturates these receptors for as long as 3 hours. Craving results when the receptor occupancy declines over time, and reducing that craving requires achieving virtually complete receptor saturation.[48–51]

The USPHS 2008 update of the Treating Tobacco Use and Dependence clinical practice guidelines categorizes pharmacotherapy into first-line and second-line medications and also addresses combinations of medications. All first-line medications seem to be of similar effectiveness. First-line medications include nicotine replacement therapy (NRT), bupropion, and varenicline (**Table 3**).[44,52] All of these medications were found to be effective first-line medications in the guideline's meta-analyses. Second-line medications include clonidine and nortriptyline. There is significant evidence that the odds of a smoker quitting are increased by using a pharmacologic approach.[44,52]

Regardless of the level of physical addiction or the number of cigarettes smoked daily, the guideline recommends that all patients attempting to quit should be encouraged to at least try one or more of the effective pharmacotherapy agents. The goal of cessation pharmacotherapy is to alleviate or diminish the symptoms of nicotine withdrawal and diminish the urge to smoke.

Nicotine Replacement Therapy

NRT was the first proven effective medication for the treatment of nicotine dependence and remains a first-line pharmacotherapy in the management of nicotine withdrawal symptoms.[53] NRT makes it easier to abstain from tobacco by replacing, at least partially, the nicotine obtained from tobacco and to quash the nicotine withdrawal symptoms and cravings seen on discontinuation of tobacco use.

NRT is available in five modalities, including the long-acting nicotine patch and the short-acting gum, lozenge, inhaler, and nasal spray (see **Table 3**). All NRTs are nicotinic acetylcholine receptor agonists but compared with smoking a cigarette, the nicotine by NRT products is delivered much more slowly and at a lower dose and do not reproduce the rapid and high levels of nicotine achieved through inhalation of cigarette smoke. Therefore, amelioration of symptoms of nicotine withdrawal is not absolute and dose adjustment is required. The transdermal patch system offers a continuous release of nicotine over 15 or 24 hours depending on the brand, whereas the oral formulations are short-acting, so the dose can be self-titrated, thus time-adjusted to the patient's needs.

A Cochrane review of 132 trials with more than 40,000 patients found that all forms of NRT increase quit rates by 50% to 70%.[54] Combination NRT (eg, the patch plus the gum) may further improve quit rates. The efficacies of the various forms of NRT are generally similar but compliance with the various delivery forms may be the limiting factor. One study comparing four forms of NRT found comparable 12-week abstinence rates (20%–24%) but compliance varied: 11% with the inhaler, 15% with the nasal spray, 38% with the gum, and 82% with the patch.[55]

It seems possible to improve the efficacy of NRT by combining the transdermal patch with an oral formulation that permits ad libitum nicotine delivery.[56] NRT is typically started the day of the quit date, although precessation treatment is considered safe and it may be advantageous for smokers to try NRT before the stress of quitting to determine which agent or agents are preferable. The PHS prescribing guideline does not officially recommend using NRT while smoking; however, it is becoming more common for patients to be started on NRT before their quit date.

Physicians who prescribe NRT for tobacco dependence should individualize the dose and duration of treatment based on the patient's response including the subjective relief of withdrawal symptoms and cravings. If NRT is selected for treatment, a combination therapy of nicotine patches and short-acting NRT is usually preferred over monotherapy with a short-acting NRT product. Short-acting NRT is best used for the acute management of nicotine withdrawal symptoms and cravings in combination with longer-acting medications, such as nicotine patches, bupropion, or varenicline. Nicotine doses

Table 3
Pharmacologic smoking cessation aids

	Patches	Gum	Lozenge	Nasal Spray	Inhaler	Zyban (Bupropion)	Chantix (Varenicline)
Duration of therapy	12 wk or more, then can use as needed	12 wk or more, then can use as needed	12 wk or more, then can use as needed	12 wk or more, then can use as needed	12 wk or more, then can use as needed	12 wk or more; start 1–2 wk before quitting	12 wk or more; start 1–2 wk before quitting
Dose	21 mg if smoke a pack a day, 14 mg if smoke half a pack a day; 7 mg if smoke 4–5 cigarettes a day (can double up on patches or use patch with another system if smoke more than a pack a day)	4 mg if smoke a pack a day, 2 mg if smoke less than a pack a day – chew at least 1 piece for every 2 cigarettes smoked	4 mg if smoke a pack or more a day, 2 mg if smoke less than a pack a day – can use 1 lozenge every 1–2 h	Dose once or twice an hour (nor more than 48 sprays in 24 h)	6–12 cartridges a day	Bupropion SR: One 150-mg tablet every morning for 3 d, then one 150-mg table twice a day at least 8 h apart on Day 4 and thereafter Bupropion extended release: one 150-mg tablet every morning for 1 wk, then one 300-mg tablet every morning thereafter	One 0.5-mg tablet for 3 d, then one 0.5-mg tablet twice a day for 4 d, then one 1-mg tablet twice a day thereafter; take each tablet after a meal and with a full glass of water
Pros	Very easy to use; automatically gives the right dose in 24-h period; helps with early morning cravings	Easy to regulate dose; can help prevent overeating; can provide extra help at difficult moments	Easy to regulate dose; can help prevent overeating; can provide extra help at difficult moments	Gives fast relief and easy to adjust dose	Helps keep hands and mouth busy, easy to regulate, could help prevent overeating	Good short-term research results; easy to use; noticeable reduction in number and severity of urges to smoke	Better than Zyban short- and long-term research results; easy to use; noticeable reduction in number and severity of urges to smoke; no cigarette "reward"
Cons	Can cause vivid dreams at night; not orally gratifying; small possibility of skin reaction	Difficult to use correctly (nothing to drink 20 min prior; chew and park)	Difficult to use correctly (nothing to drink 20 min prior; let dissolve slowly)	May cause nasal irritation	Feels and looks like a cigarette; very conspicuous method	Possible sleep disruption and can cause dry mouth	Possible nausea, vivid dreams; Possible association with increased depression or suicidal ideation

should be increased for patients experiencing pronounced withdrawal symptoms, such as irritability, anxiety, loss of concentration, or cravings.

Nicotine gum is available as an over-the-counter product, in 2- and 4-mg doses. Patients should be instructed in its proper use to "chew and park" and to avoid acidic beverages that lower the intraoral pH and thereby reduce nicotine absorption. Nicotine gum can be used as monotherapy or in combination with other NRT or bupropion.

The nicotine lozenge is available as an over-the-counter product. The nicotine lozenge is available in 2- and 4-mg doses, with the latter indicated for use in high-dependence smokers (ie, time to first cigarette of the day of <30 minutes after arising). The method of delivery (transbuccal) is similar to that of nicotine gum, and it can be used alone or in combination with other NRT or bupropion.

Nicotine nasal spray delivers nicotine directly to the nasal mucosa and has been observed to be effective for achieving smoking abstinence as monotherapy. This device delivers nicotine more rapidly than other therapeutic nicotine replacement delivery systems and reduces withdrawal symptoms more quickly than nicotine gum.[52] The reduction in withdrawal symptoms may be partially attributable to the rapidity with which nicotine is absorbed from the nasal mucosa.

The nicotine vapor inhaler has also been shown to be effective as monotherapy for increasing smoking abstinence.[57] The device delivers nicotine in vapor form that is absorbed across the oral mucosa. Although the device is called an inhaler, this is a misnomer because little of the nicotine vapor reaches the pulmonary alveoli, even with deep inhalations.

Nicotine patch therapy delivers a steady dose of nicotine for 24 hours after a single application. The once-daily dosing requires little effort on the part of the patient, which enhances compliance. Nicotine patches are available without a prescription in doses of 7, 14, and 21 mg. In nearly every randomized clinical trial performed to date, the nicotine patch has been shown to be effective compared with placebo, usually with a doubling of the smoking abstinence rate.[54]

Most patients use NRT for 4 to 8 weeks but it is safe for longer use if needed to maintain smoking abstinence. The optimal length of treatment has not been determined but longer-term treatment (>14 weeks) seems to provide benefit over standard lengths of treatment when combining nicotine patches and nicotine gum.[43] Furthermore, long-term treatment of up to 6 months with triple combination therapy (nicotine patches, bupropion, and nicotine vapor inhaler) seems superior to standard-dose nicotine patch therapy given over a 10-week period.[43] For the best chance at success with these therapies, they may be used in combination and should be dose-appropriate based on the patient's need.

Label Warning and Contraindications for NRT Products

The labeling on NRT products still instructs tobacco users to consult their physician if there is a history of heart disease, ulcers, hypertension, pregnancy, or breast-feeding. This is despite the fact there is a documented lack of an association between NRT and acute cardiovascular events even in patients who continue to smoke while on the patch. Because trials specifically excluded patients with unstable angina, serious arrhythmias, and recent myocardial infarction, the Clinical Practice Guideline recommends that NRT be used with caution among patients in the immediate (within 2 weeks) post–myocardial infarction period, those with serious arrhythmias, and those with serious or worsening angina because of a lack of safety data. Despite this caution, it is widely believed that the risks of NRT in patients with cardiovascular disease are minimal relative to the risks of continued tobacco use. The guideline recommends use of NRT in pregnancy if other therapies have failed. Clearly, the fetus is exposed to significantly less nicotine with NRT than with smoking and most importantly is not exposed to carbon monoxide, carcinogens, and toxins from cigarettes.

Nonnicotine Medications

There are two nonnicotine medications specifically developed to help adults quit smoking that have been proved to be the most effective pharmacotherapy treatment: bupropion and varenicline (see **Table 3**). Varenicline is considered more effective based on randomized trials.[58,59] The US Food and Drug Administration (FDA) has issued boxed warnings for both drugs because of reports of increased risks of psychiatric symptoms and suicide. Given the well-established link between smoking and psychiatric disease, there is no easy way to determine whether or not these adverse events are directly related to the medications. Unfortunately, these warnings may deter clinicians from discussing or prescribing bupropion and varenicline.

Bupropion (Wellbutrin/Zyban)

Bupropion sustained release (SR) was the first nonnicotinic medication approved by the FDA for smoking cessation. It has been on the market as an antidepressant since the 1980s. Bupropion is known to inhibit the reuptake of norepinephrine and dopamine, and it is a nicotinic acetylcholine receptor antagonist. The exact mechanism for its efficacy in smoking cessation is unknown and likely multifactorial.

Bupropion has been shown to increase smoking cessation rates from 12% in patients using placebo to 23% in those using bupropion.[60] In addition, studies have suggested that a combined approach with bupropion plus a nicotine patch may be even more effective. The dose of bupropion is 150 mg of the SR form starting with one tablet per day, preferably on waking, for 3 days, then increasing to one table twice daily. The doses should be separated by at least 8 hours with the second dose as far away from bedtime as possible. The 2008 USPHS Guideline recommends the combined use of bupropion SR and NRT for at least 3 months.[45]

Unlike other antidepressants, bupropion typically does not cause weight gain (and may suppress it) or sexual dysfunction so it may be especially of interest to those patients concerned about weight gain when quitting smoking. Bupropion extended release is also available for once-a-day dosing. Treatment with bupropion with either dosing is typically initiated 1 to 2 weeks before quit date.

Varenicline

The most recent nonnicotine medication is varenicline (Chantix), a partial agonist selective for a specific nicotine receptor subtype. Varenicline was approved in by the FDA in 2006 and introduced in the updated 2008 guideline. It is a partial agonist at the $cx4\beta2$ neuronal nicotinic acetylcholine receptor causing a sustained moderate level of dopamine release, which is thought to reduce withdrawal symptoms. It also acts as an antagonist at the $cx4\beta2$ neuronal nicotinic acetylcholine receptor, which may inhibit the rewarding effects of nicotine and reduce or eliminate satisfaction relating to smoking. There are currently no known contraindications to varenicline therapy. It should be used in caution in patients with chronic kidney disease and the dose should be lowered by half in patients with creatinine clearance less than 30 mL/min.

Evidence suggests that using varenicline can appreciably increase quit rates compared with bupropion and placebo.[58,59,61] Varenicline has demonstrated superior efficacy compared with placebo in multiple clinical trials, several of which were conducted before regulatory approval in 2006 in the United States and Europe. Meta-analyses have confirmed the increased efficacy of varenicline at the dosage of 2 mg/day during a 12-week treatment on smoking quit rates compared with placebo and also with bupropion. Varenicline has also been shown to perform better than treatment with the transdermal NRT patch. The combination of varenicline with NRT or bupropion seems safe and the latter may result in better quit rates than monotherapy.[62,63]

Pivotal trials in healthy smokers comparing varenicline at a dose of 1 mg twice daily with placebo or bupropion SR have demonstrated that varenicline is more effective, with end of treatment (12 weeks) continuous smoking abstinence rates of 44% versus 30% for bupropion SR and 18% for placebo.[64,65] An additional 12 weeks of varenicline has been shown to be effective in maintaining smoking abstinence in smokers who had stopped smoking after 12 weeks of open-label varenicline treatment.

Varenicline is supplied in a "Starting Month Pack" and a "Continuing Month Pack." The Starting Pack begins with 0.5 mg daily for 3 days, followed by 0.5 mg twice daily for 4 days. The target quit date is Day 8 when the maintenance dose of 1 mg twice daily begins. The initial treatment period should be at least 12 weeks (one starting pack plus two continuing packs). The decision to continue past 12 weeks should be individualized, keeping in mind that higher quit rates are seen with longer duration of treatment.

Combination Therapy

For the first time, the 2008 clinical practice guideline update assessed the relative effectiveness of cessation medications and multiple combinations of medications were shown to be effective. These comparisons showed that two forms of pharmacotherapy, varenicline (Chantix) used alone and the combination of a long-term nicotine patch plus as-needed nicotine nasal spray or gum, produced significantly higher long-term quit rates than did the patch by itself. Combining two kinds of NRT with different types of delivery (the more rapid oral products with the slower absorbed patch) has been shown to improve quit rates.[54] More recent data suggest that aggressive regimens in the form of triple-combination therapy (inhaler, patch, and nasal spray) in combination with bupropion are a safe and effective treatment.[66] Combination therapy with medications from different classes, including the patch with bupropion, has shown improved efficacy over monotherapy. Preliminary data also suggest varenicline in combination with NRT or bupropion may be efficacious and well tolerated.[62] However, future controlled trials are required to confirm these findings. Combination therapy is "off label" use but now it is definitively medically sanctioned.

Relapse

Relapse should be seen as a probable event, especially within the first 3 months of the quit attempt. Even among patients who succeed in quitting for extended periods, relapse occurs in 75% of first-time quitters.[42] Relapse is usually preceded by slips, defined as taking one puff or smoking an entire cigarette. If slips occur for more than 7 days, the patient is considered to be a regular smoker again. Smokers who have been abstinent for 24 to 48 hours have made a serious attempt at quitting and are the most vulnerable to relapse.[67] Smokers who experience a lapse in the first few weeks of cessation are also at high risk for returning to smoking. Most relapse (75%) happens in conjunction with alcohol consumption, whereas 50% of relapse occurs if living, socializing, or working with other smokers.[41] The most common thought preceding a slip is, "I can have just one."

Smokers who are unable to quit on their target quit date but eventually quit using pharmacotherapy seem to benefit from additional 12 weeks of therapy. Smokers taking varenicline have the most success quitting compared with those taking other first-line pharmacotherapy for treating tobacco dependence.

RECOMMENDATIONS AND BEST PRACTICES FOR SMOKING CESSATION

The updated Clinical Practice guideline[45] analyses suggest that a wide variety of clinicians can effectively implement cessation strategies. Cessation interventions as brief as 3 minutes can significantly increase cessation quit rates. Successful tobacco abstinence not only reduces general medical costs in the short-term but also reduces the number of future hospitalizations. Smoking cessation intervention is extremely cost-effective relative to other common disease prevention interventions and medical treatments,[44] such as the treatment of hypertension and hypercholesterolemia, and preventive screening interventions, such as periodic mammography and Papanicolaou tests.

A practical way to ensure assessment of tobacco consumption is to consider tobacco use as "the new vital sign" obtained and recorded by the office staff who records other routine vital signs. Once identified, all smokers should receive clear, concise, and simple advice to quit (see **Tables 1** and **2**). Smokers need assistance in developing a plan for quitting that includes a quit date, practical counseling help, and effective medications.

A brief (3 minute) counseling session should focus on two key questions. First the clinician should ask if the patient has knowledge about how to quit. If the patient responds to this question affirmatively, the clinician should set a quit date and recommend a cessation pharmacotherapy. Few health interventions have such overwhelming evidence of effectiveness as smoking cessation medications. The seven first-line FDA-approved therapies reliably increase long-term smoking abstinence rates (see **Table 3**). All approximately double the rate of cessation compared with placebo.

SUMMARY

Although providing evidence-based treatment for tobacco-dependent patients can be a challenge for the busy surgeon, it is a realistic clinical endeavor. In contrast to two decades ago, tobacco users are now able to select from many treatment options. It is well established that the use of approved medications for cessation at least doubles the odds of quitting and medications should be coupled with approaches that promote behavioral changes, such as advice from a healthcare provider.

The 2008 clinical practice guideline presents more compelling evidence for the efficacy and cost effectiveness of treatment for tobacco use and dependence. For clinicians, the guideline offers four key conclusions: (1) tobacco dependence is a chronic remitting and relapsing condition and repeated attempts to quit should be encouraged for all smokers at every opportunity; (2) counseling as brief as 3 minutes is an effective treatment for tobacco dependence; (3) a larger number of effective medications and medication combinations are currently available and should be used for all smokers who are motivated to quit; and (4) of all the first-line medications provided as monotherapy, varenicline seems to have the greatest efficacy after 3 to 6 months. Clinicians should take every opportunity to encourage smoking cessation and provide effective treatment.

The most important message professionals can communicate to tobacco users is that it is never too late to quit. Even for long-term smokers, quitting smoking carries major and immediate health benefits for men and women of all ages. Benefits apply to healthy people and to those already suffering from smoking-related disease. For United States surgeons, the potential benefits far outweigh the investment. If all of the estimated

10 million smokers undergoing elective surgery this year were offered a smoking cessation intervention that succeeded in only 25% of cases, 2 million complications would be avoided.[25] Global fiscal implications are even more staggering because up to 70 million adult smokers undergo major surgery annually. As third-party payers and hospitals know, complications escalate healthcare costs. It is time for physicians, surgeons, hospitals, and payers to embrace routine preoperative smoking-cessation practices.

REFERENCES

1. World Health Organization. WHO Report on the Global Tobacco Epidemic, 2008: The MPOWER Package 2008. Geneva (Switzerland): World Health Organization; 2008.
2. Action on Smoking and Health. Essential information on tobacco and the developing world. London: ASH; 2007. Available at: http//www.ash.org.uk/files/documents/ASH_126pdf. Accessed May 30, 2011.
3. U.S. Department of Health and Human Services. Health, United States 2005. With chartbook on trends in the health of Americans. Hyattsville (MD): Centers for Disease Control and Prevention, National Center for Health Statistics; 2005.
4. Schroeder SA. Tobacco control in the wake of the 1998 Master Settlement Agreement. N Engl J Med 2004;350:293–301.
5. Centers for Disease Control and Prevention. Cigarette smoking among adults—United States, 2004. MMWR Morb Mortal Wkly Rep 2005;54:1121–4.
6. Herman AI. Sofuoglu. Curr Psychiatry Rep 2010;12: 433–40.
7. Centers for Disease Control and Prevention. Best practices for comprehensive tobacco control programs—2007. Atlanta (GA): US Department of Health and Human Services, Centers for Disease Control and Prevention, National Center for Chronic Disease Prevention and Health Promotion, Office on Smoking and Health; 2007.
8. Tobacco epidemic: much more than a health issue. WHO FACT Sheet No. 154. Geneva (Switzerland): World Health Organization; 1998.
9. Chaloupka FJ. Curbing the epidemic: governments and the economics of tobacco control. Washington, DC: The World Bank; 1999.
10. World Health Organization. WHO Framework Convention on Tobacco Control. Geneva (Switzerland): World Health Organization; 2003.
11. Mokad AH, Marks JS, Stroup DF, et al. Actual causes of death in the United States 2000. JAMA 2004;10:1238–45.
12. McIvor A, Kayser J, Assad JM, et al. Best practices for smoking cessation interventions in primary care. Can Respir J 2009;16:129–34.
13. Alberg AI, Samet JM. Epidemiology of lung cancer. Chest 2003;123:215.
14. Boffetta P, Tubiana M, Hill C, et al. The causes of cancer in France. Ann Oncol 2009;20:550–5.
15. International Agency for Research on Cancer. Tobacco smoke and involuntary smoking. IARC monographs on the evaluation of carcinogenic risk to humans. Lyon (France): IARC; 2004. p. 83.
16. Cooley ME, Emmons KM, Haddad R, et al. Patient-reported receipt of and interest in smoking-cessation interventions after the diagnosis of cancer. Cancer 2011;117:2961–9.
17. White JR. Treating nicotine addiction with OTC products. US Pharmacist 2007;32:18–21.
18. US Department of Health and Human Services. The Health Benefits of Smoking Cessation. A report from the Surgeon General. Washington: US Department of Health and Human Services, CDC publication 90–8416; 1990.
19. Cox LS, Patten CA, Ebbert JO, et al. Tobacco use outcomes among patients with lung cancer treated for nicotine dependence. J Clin Oncol 2002;20: 3461–9.
20. Xu J, Huang H, Pan C, et al. B nicotine inhibits apoptosis induced by cisplatin in human oral cancer cells. Int J Oral Maxillofac Surg 2007;36:739–44.
21. Baser S, Shannon V, Eapan G, et al. Smoking cessation after diagnosis of lung cancer is associated with a beneficial effect on performance status. Chest 2006;130:1784–90.
22. Richardson GE, Tucker MA, Venzon DJ, et al. Smoking cessation after successful treatment of small cell lung cancer is associated with fewer smoking-related secondary primary cancers. Ann Intern Med 1993;119:383–90.
23. Delgado M, Medina M, Martinez G, et al. A prospective study of tobacco smoking as a predictor of complications in general surgery. Infect Control Hosp Epidemiol 2003;24:36–43.
24. Thomsen T, Tonnesen H, Moller AM. Effect of preoperative smoking cessation interventions on postoperative complications and smoking cessation. Br J Surg 2009;96:451–61.
25. Mills E, Eyawo O, Lockhart I, et al. Smoking cessation reduces postoperative complications: a systematic review and meta-analysis. Am J Med 2011;124: 144–54.
26. Myers K, Hajek P, Hinds C, et al. Stopping smoking shortly before surgery and perioperative complications. A systematic review and meta-analysis. Arch Intern Med 2011;171(11):983–9.
27. Slatore CG, Au DH, Hollingworth W. Cost-effectiveness of a smoking cessation program implemented at the time of surgery for lung cancer. J Thorac Oncol 2009;4:499–504.
28. Waller LL, Weaver KE, Petty WJ, et al. Effects of continued tobacco use during treatment of lung

cancer. Expert Rev Anticancer Ther 2010;10: 1569–75.

29. Wolfenden L, Wiggers J, Knight J, et al. A programme for reducing smoking in pre-operative surgical patients: randomised controlled trial. Anaesthesia 2005;60:172–9.

30. Sardari NP, Weyler J, Colpaert C, et al. Prognostic value of smoking status in operated non-small cell lung cancer. Lung Cancer 2005;47:351–9.

31. Bluman LG, Mosca L, Newman N, et al. Preoperative smoking habits and postoperative pulmonary complications. Chest 1998;113:883–9.

32. Warner MA, Offord KP, Warner ME, et al. Role of preoperative cessation of smoking and other factors in postoperative pulmonary complications: a blinded prospective study of coronary artery bypass patients. Mayo Clin Proc 1989;64:609–16.

33. Nakagawa M, Tanaka H, Tsukuma H, et al. Relationship between the duration of the preoperative smoke-free period and the incidence of postoperative complications after pulmonary surgery. Chest 2001;120:705–10.

34. Groth SS, Whitson BA, Kuskowski MA, et al. Impact of preoperative smoking status on postoperative complication rates and pulmonary function test results 1-year following resection for non-small cell lung cancer. Lung Cancer 2009;64:352–7.

35. Theadom A, Cropley M. Effects of perioperative smoking cessation on the incidence and risk of intra-operative and postoperative complications in adult smokers: a systematic review. Tob Control 2006;15: 352–8.

36. Lindstrom D, Azodi OS, Wladis A, et al. Effects of perioperative smoking cessation intervention on postoperative complications. A randomized trial. Ann Surg 2008;248:739–45.

37. Barrera R, Shi W, Amar D, et al. Smoking and timing of cessation: impact on pulmonary complications after thoracotomy. Chest 2005;127:1977–83.

38. Moller A, Tonnesen H. Risk reduction: perioperative smoking intervention. Best Pract Res Clin Anaesthesiol 2006;20:237–48.

39. Mason DP, Subramanian S, Nowicki ER, et al. Impact of smoking cessation before resection of lung cancer: a Society of Thoracic Surgeons general thoracic surgery database study. Ann Thorac Surg 2009;88:362–71.

40. Thomsen T, Villebro N, Møller AM. Interventions for preoperative smoking cessation. Cochrane Database Syst Rev 2010;7:CD002294.

41. Yudkin P, Hey K, Roberts S, et al. Abstinence from smoking eight years after participation in randomized controlled trial of nicotine patch. BMJ 2003; 327(7405):28–9.

42. Hughes JR, Keely J, Naud S. Shape of the relapse curve and long-term abstinence among untreated smokers. Addiction 2004;99(1):29–38.

43. Steinberg MB, Schmelzer AC, Richardson DL, et al. The case for treating tobacco dependence as a chronic disease. Ann Intern Med 2008;148(7): 554–6.

44. Fiore MC, Jaen CR, Baker TB, et al. Treating tobacco use and dependence: 2008 update. Washington, DC: US Department of Health and Human Services, Public Health Service; 2008.

45. The Clinical Practice Guideline Treating Tobacco Use and Dependence 2008 Update Panel, Liaisons, and Staff. A clinical practice guideline for treating tobacco use and dependence: 2008 update. A U.S. Public Health Service report. Am J Prev Med 2008;35(2):158–76.

46. Zillich AJ, Corelli RL, Hudmon KS. Smoking cessation for the busy clinician. The Rx Consultant 2007; 16(8):1–8.

47. Stead LF, Lancaster T, Perera R. Telephone counseling for smoking cessation. Cochrane Database Syst Rev 2003;1:CD002850.

48. Rose JE, Behm FM, Westman EC, et al. Arterial nicotine kinetics during cigarette smoking and intravenous nicotine administration: implications for addiction. Drug Alcohol Depend 1999;56(2): 99–107.

49. Picciotto MR, Zoli M, Rimondini R, et al. Acetylcholine receptors containing the β2 subunit are involved in the reinforcing properties of nicotine. Nature 1998; 391:173–7.

50. Pontieri FE, Tanda G, Orzi F, et al. Effects of nicotine on the nucleus accumbens and similarity to those of addictive drugs. Nature 1996;382(6588):255–7.

51. Nisell M, Nomikos GG, Svensson TH. Systemic nicotine-induced dopamine release in the rat nucleus accumbens is regulated by nicotinic receptors in the ventral tegmental area. Synapse 1994; 16(1):36–44.

52. Drugs for tobacco dependence. Treat Guidel Med Lett 2008;6:61–6.

53. Edens E, Massa A, Petrakis I. Novel pharmacological approaches to drug abuse treatment. Curr Top Behav Neurosci 2010;3:343–86.

54. Stead LF, Perera R, Bullen C, et al. Nicotine replacement therapy for smoking cessation. Cochrane Database Syst Rev 2008;1:CD000145.

55. Hajek P, West R, Foulds J, et al. Randomized comparative trial of nicotine polarilex, a transdermal patch, nasal spray, and an inhaler. Arch Intern Med 1999;159:2033–8.

56. Sweeney CT, Fant RV, Gagerstrom KO, et al. Combination nicotine replacement therapy for smoking cessation: rationale, efficacy and tolerability. CNS Drugs 2001;15(6):453–67.

57. Bolliger CT, Zellweger JP, Danielsson T, et al. Clinical pharmacokinetics of nasal nicotine delivery. A review and comparison to other nicotine systems. Clin Pharmacokinet 1996;31:65–80.

58. Hays JT, Ebbert JO, Sood A. Efficacy and safety of varenicline for smoking cessation. Am J Med 2008; 121(Suppl 1):S32–42.

59. Nides M, Gover ED, Reus VI, et al. Varenicline versus bupropion SR or placebo for smoking cessation: a pooled analysis. Am J Health Behav 2008; 32(6):664–75.

60. Hurt RD, Sachs DPI, Glover ED, et al. A comparison of sustained-released bupropion and placebo for smoking cessation. N Engl J Med 1997;337(17): 1195–202.

61. Cahill K, Stead LF, Lancester T. Nicotine receptor partial agonists for smoking cessation. Cochrane Database Syst Rev 2010;12:CD006103.

62. Ebbert JO, Burke MV, Hays JT, et al. Combination treatment with varenicline and nicotine replacement therapy. Nicotine Tob Res 2009; 11(5):572–6.

63. Ebbert JO, Croghan IT, Sood A, et al. Varenicline and bupropion sustained-release combination therapy for smoking cessation. Nicotine Tob Res 2009;11(3):234–9.

64. Gonzales D, Rennard SI, Mides M, et al. Varenicline, an alpja4beta2nicotinic acetylcholine receptor partial agonist, vs sustained-release bupropion and placebo for smoking cessation: a randomized controlled trial. JAMA 2006;296:47–55.

65. Jornby JE, Hays JT, Rigotti NA, et al. Efficacy of varenicline, an $\alpha4\beta2$ nicotinic acetylcholine receptor partial agonist, vs placebo or sustained-release bupropion for smoking cessation: a randomized controlled trial. JAMA 2006;296:56–63.

66. Steinberg MV, Greenhaus S, Schmelzer AC, et al. Triple-combination pharmacotherapy for medically ill smokers: a randomized trial. Ann Intern Med 2009;150(7):447–54.

67. Fiore MC, Bailey WC, Cohen SJ, et al. Treating tobacco use and dependence. Clinical practice guideline. Rockville (MD): US Department of Health and Human Services, Public Health Service; 2000.

Prophylaxis and Management of Atrial Fibrillation After General Thoracic Surgery

Robert E. Merritt, MD[a], Joseph B. Shrager, MD[a,b],*

KEYWORDS

- Atrial arrhythmia • Thoracic surgery • Anticoagulation

Atrial fibrillation (AF) is the most common arrhythmia that affects patients following general thoracic surgical procedures. After pulmonary resection and esophagectomy, AF occurs in between 12% and 44% of patients.[1] It is defined as a supraventricular tachyarrhythmia characterized by uncoordinated atrial activity with resultant ineffective mechanical function.[2] The ECG demonstrates irregular low-amplitude oscillations with the absence of regular P waves. Atrial rates can often exceed 300 beats/min, and conduction through the atrioventricular node can reach 200 beats/min. AF in the medical population is most commonly associated with conditions such as hypertension, hyperthyroidism, alcohol abuse, mitral valve disease, coronary artery disease, and pulmonary embolism.

Patients with postoperative AF have been shown to have increased lengths of stay, increased mortality, and increased hospital charges.[1] Thus, effective prophylaxis and prompt, successful treatment of AF is an important goal. This article is a review of the current management recommendations for AF in patients undergoing general thoracic surgical procedures. These recommendations are adapted from the Society of Thoracic Surgeons (STS) Clinical Practice Guidelines on this topic (www.sts.org/resources-publications).[3] The concepts reviewed are prophylaxis of AF, treatment of AF by rate control, treatment of AF by rhythm control, and the role of anticoagulation. This article attempts to provide a framework for general thoracic surgeons to use to prevent and manage AF, and to minimize the morbidity and costs associated with this common arrhythmia.

CAUSES AND RISK FACTORS

AF tends to arise in the substrate of abnormal atrial tissue that is affected by inflammation or fibrosis.[2,4] The onset of AF usually requires a trigger, which may be an alteration in automaticity, a change in atrial wall tension, or the development of an atrial ectopic focus.[5] Reentrant circuits that collide within the walls of the atria are another cause.[6] Although the electrical mechanisms of AF remain incompletely understood, the influences on AF relevant to patients undergoing thoracic surgery include age, myocardial ischemia, volume overload, elevated norepinephrine levels with changes in autonomic tone, and trauma to the atria or pulmonary veins.[7] The region of the pulmonary veins, which obviously are in the

The authors have nothing to disclose.

[a] Division of Thoracic Surgery, Department of Cardiothoracic Surgery, Stanford University School of Medicine, 300 Pasteur Drive, Stanford, CA 94305, USA

[b] Division of Thoracic Surgery, VA Palo Alto Health Care System, 3801 Miranda Avenue, Palo Alto, CA 94304, USA

* Corresponding author. Stanford Medical Center, 2nd Floor Falk Building, 300 Pasteur Drive, Stanford, CA 94305.

E-mail address: Shrager@stanford.edu

field of many general thoracic procedures, provide one common locus for the initiation of AF.[8]

The risk factors for postoperative AF include advanced age, male gender, extent of pulmonary resection and esophageal resection, history of congestive heart failure, COPD, preoperative arrhythmias, prior thoracotomy, intraoperative blood transfusion, and procedures associated with dissection around the atria.[1,9–11] Reportedly, the highest rates of postoperative AF occur after pneumonectomy and lung transplantation, which involve significant dissection around the pulmonary veins and the mediastinum.[1,12,13] The rate of postoperative AF in recent large series of thoracoscopic lobectomy range from 2.9% to 10%.[14–16] A recent propensity-matched analysis from the STS database[15] demonstrates a significantly lower rate of postoperative AF in a thoracoscopic lobectomy cohort compared with an open lobectomy cohort (7.26% vs 11.48%; $P = .0004$). The exact explanation for this observation is not known, but it may be related either to the apparently lower inflammatory response in thoracoscopic lobectomy patients or to the reduced hilar-mediastinal dissection in those patients.

Prophylaxis of Postoperative AF

Recommendations for pharmacologic prophylaxis of postoperative AF are summarized in **Table 1**.

CONTINUATION OF PREOPERATIVE BETA BLOCKERS

Perhaps the simplest way to avoid AF in postoperative patients is to promptly resume preoperative beta blockers that a patient had been taking. There are randomized, prospective data demonstrating that beta blocker withdrawal produces an increase in postoperative AF following elective cardiac surgery. Reports of a "propranolol withdrawal syndrome" leading to increased rates of arrhythmias and coronary events first appeared in the 1970s, when there had been a recommendation that patients preparing for elective coronary surgery have beta blockers stopped before the operation.[17,18] As an example of one of several, randomized studies establishing this phenomenon,[19] AF occurred in 39% of a beta blocker withdrawal group and 17% of a postoperative beta blocker group ($P<.02$). In another study,

Table 1
Pharmacologic prophylaxis of postoperative AF

Agent	Level of Evidence	Recommendation
Beta-Blocker	Class I	Patients taking beta-blockers before GTS should have beta-blockade continued in the postoperative period
Diltiazem	Class IIa	Diltiazem prophylaxis is reasonable in most patients undergoing major pulmonary resection who are not taking a beta-blocker preoperatively. As with beta-blockers, some patients receiving diltiazem prophylaxis may develop hypotension, so dose reduction or other pressure-elevating therapies may be required
Amiodarone	Class IIa	Amiodarone prophylaxis is reasonable to reduce the incidence of AF following GTS (excluding pneumonectomy), according to strict dosing regimens. For patients undergoing pulmonary lobectomy, the recommended dosage is 1050 mg via continuous infusion over the first 24 h following surgery (43.75 mg/h), followed by 400 mg orally bid for 6 d. For patients undergoing esophagectomy, the recommended dose is continuous IV infusion at a rate of 43.75 mg/h (1050 mg qd) for 4 d
Magnesium	Class IIa	Magnesium supplementation is reasonable to augment the prophylactic effects of other medications
Beta-Blocker	Class IIb	It may be reasonable to initiate new beta-blockers as prophylaxis against postoperative AF following GTS, but their use is more limited by side effects than is Diltiazem
Amiodarone	Class III	Amiodarone is not recommended, outside of clinical studies, in those undergoing pneumonectomy, until additional data addressing its potential toxicity in this setting are available

Abbreviation: GTS, general thoracic surgery.

mean norepinephrine levels were found to be significantly higher in those patients receiving preoperative beta blockers (which were withdrawn postoperatively) compared with those not receiving these drugs.[20] These increased norepinephrine levels may be a mechanism for the increased incidence of postoperative AF when beta blockers are discontinued.

Because episodes of hypotension are common after general thoracic surgical operations (particularly in patients with epidural analgesia), it is recommended to adjust the preoperative dose of beta blocker downward but not to withdraw beta blockers completely. Specifically, if epidural analgesia is being used, the authors recommend that preoperative beta blockade be restarted early postoperatively at one-half the equivalent pharmacologic dosage. The dosage can typically be increased back to the full preoperative dosage when the epidural catheter is removed. Hold parameters should always be written based on minimal tolerable blood pressure and heart rate. If bradycardia or hypotension occurs, the dosage can be further reduced and/or individual doses held.

CALCIUM-CHANNEL BLOCKER PROPHYLAXIS

The authors believe—and the STS *Guidelines* recommend—that patients undergoing substantial pulmonary resections who were not taking beta blockers preoperatively (in whom beta blockers, therefore, would be resumed postoperatively) should have prophylactic diltiazem begun in the early postoperative period.

In an attempt to minimize the risk of postoperative AF, thoracic surgeons have studied several prophylactic antiarrhythmic therapies. A meta-analysis by Sedrakyan and colleagues[21] reviewed 11 randomized, controlled, clinical trials (n = 1294) that evaluated the efficacy of prophylactic medications in reducing atrial tachyarrhythmia after general thoracic surgery. Calcium-channel blockers reduced the risk of atrial tachyarrhythmias in four of the clinical studies with a relative risk (RR) of 0.50 and a 95% confidence interval (CI) of 0.34 to 0.73. Newly initiated beta blockers reduced the risk of AF in two of the studies (RR 0.40; 95% CI, 0.17–0.95). However, the risk of developing pulmonary edema and other adverse events was higher in patients who received new beta blocker therapy. Digitalis was found to actually increase the rate of postoperative AF (RR of 1.25–2.92). The efficacy of flecainide and amiodarone were uncertain in two separate trials in the meta-analysis. The small trial (n = 30) that investigated flecainide did

demonstrate a reduction in arrhythmic events, but the trial was too small to address the endpoints of the meta-analysis. The amiodarone trial demonstrated a significant reduction in AF, but there were two mortalities related to adult respiratory distress syndrome (ARDS) in the amiodarone cohort (see later discussion). The patients in the meta-analysis seemed to be reasonably representative of a typical general thoracic surgery practice. The average age of subjects was 63.2 years, pneumonectomies were performed in 20.9% of the cases, and the postoperative rate of AF in the placebo groups was in the range of 16% to 26%.

Calcium channel blockers are effective atrioventricular nodal blockers and are known to reduce pulmonary vascular resistance. In addition, calcium channel blockers are not associated with the potential bronchospastic side effects of beta blockers. This advantage makes calcium blockers attractive for use in patients undergoing lung resections, many of whom have baseline pulmonary dysfunction. Five randomized, double-blind, controlled trials compared the efficacy of calcium channel blockers to placebo or another treatment in the prophylaxis of postoperative AF in patients undergoing general thoracic surgical procedures.[22–26] The earliest report of the ability of calcium channel blockers to prevent postoperative AF following general thoracic surgery was a small, randomized, placebo-controlled trial by Lindgren and colleagues.[23] Twelve patients undergoing thoracotomy for pulmonary resection were given a continuous infusion of verapamil 0.01 mg/kg/h on the day of surgery, followed by an oral dose of 80 mg three times a day. A cohort of 13 patients received placebo. Postoperative AF did not occur in the verapamil group 0:12 (0%) versus 4:13 (31%) in the placebo group (P<.05). The measured end-diastolic right ventricular pressure was increased on the first postoperative day within the placebo group (P<.001) and was predictive of AF on the second day. This study contained a small population of patients; however, the results increased enthusiasm for further investigation of calcium channel blocker therapy for prevention of postoperative AF.

Van Mieghem and colleagues[24] conducted a prospective, randomized, placebo-controlled trial with 100 pneumonectomy and 200 lobectomy patients comparing verapamil and Amiodarone versus placebo for AF prophylaxis. One cohort received amiodarone, and the second cohort was given a verapamil intravenous (IV) loading dose, followed by an infusion of 0.125 mg/min for 3 days. This trial was stopped early by the investigators due to the alarming incidence of ARDS in the amiodarone cohort. Nonetheless, the investigators reported the data collected before study termination demonstrating that postoperative AF was reduced in both the amiodarone group (1:22, 0.05%) and the verapamil group (0:22, 0%), compared with a baseline rate of 22% (7:32) in the placebo group.

Amar and colleagues[22] reported a randomized, double-blind, placebo-controlled trial in 330 patients who were considered to be at high risk for postoperative AF. In this trial, patients received placebo (n = 163) or diltiazem (n = 167) as a loading dose of 0.25 mg/kg IV over 30 minutes, followed by 0.1 mg/kg/h for 18 to 24 hours, followed by oral sustained-release diltiazem 120 mg twice daily for 14 days. Diltiazem therapy was initiated immediately after the lobectomy or pneumonectomy procedures were completed. The results demonstrated that diltiazem therapy reduced the incidence of postoperative arrhythmia from 25% to 15% (P = .03) and decreased the incidence of clinically significant tachyarrhythmias from 19% to 10% (P = .02). The two cohorts did not demonstrate a difference in major postoperative complications or length of hospital stay, and no serious adverse events were attributed to diltiazem.

Further evidence in favor of calcium channel blocker prophylaxis was established in a randomized, controlled trial comparing diltiazem to digoxin.[26] Seventy patients undergoing pneumonectomy or extrapleural pneumonectomy at Memorial Sloan Kettering received either an initial dose of diltiazem 20 mg IV, followed by 10 mg IV every 4 hours for 24 to 36 hours, then 180 mg to 240 mg orally daily for 1 month (n = 35); or digoxin 1 mg IV load during the first 24 to 36 hours, followed by 0.125 to 0.25 mg orally for 1 month (n = 35). There was a concurrent prospective cohort of 40 patients who also had pneumonectomy without prophylaxis. Diltiazem significantly reduced the incidence of supraventricular dysrhythmias from 31% to 14% (P = .035). The digoxin group had postoperative AF rates similar to the untreated group.

In summary, calcium channel blockers have proven efficacy in preventing postoperative AF following pulmonary resection, with a roughly 50% reduction in incidence in high-risk patients. The most effective prophylactic therapeutic agent with the lowest incidence of adverse effects has been diltiazem. As described above, in the one placebo-controlled study specifically of diltiazem for prevention of AF after general thoracic surgery, diltiazem was administered as a loading dose of 0.25 mg/kg IV over 30 minutes, followed by 0.1 mg/kg/h for 18 to 24 hours, followed by oral sustained-release diltiazem 120 mg twice daily

for 14 days.[21] Given the ability of pulmonary resection patients to tolerate oral drugs almost immediately postoperatively and the excellent oral bioavailability of diltiazem, the authors believe it is reasonable to simplify this regimen and use shorter-acting, oral diltiazem beginning in the recovery room or on postoperative day one. An initial dose of 30 mg oral every 6 hours would be appropriate, increasing to 60 mg oral every 6 hours as tolerated. There is less solid evidence for diltiazem prophylaxis following esophagectomy, but the existing data also suggest effectiveness in this population.[27]

AMIODARONE PROPHYLAXIS

Because of the effectiveness of the class III antiarrhythmic agent amiodarone as therapy for postoperative AF, it has also been tested widely in prophylaxis against postoperative AF. This treatment strategy has been generally based on starting the amiodarone in the immediate postoperative period, and it has been evaluated in three prospective, randomized trials following pulmonary resection and following esophagectomy.[24,28,29] Van Mieghem and colleagues[24] compared amiodarone, verapamil, and placebo following lung resection. An amiodarone bolus of 150 mg IV over 2 minutes was followed by an infusion totaling 1200 mg over 24 hours for 3 postoperative days. Of the 62 patients entered into this study before it was closed, the overall incidence of AF was 3.1% in the amiodarone group versus 21.9% in the placebo group (RR, 0.14; 95% CI, 0.02–1.10). As mentioned previously, however, this trial was terminated early because of an alarmingly high incidence of ARDS (27%) in those patients who had undergone pneumonectomy and received amiodarone. The overall incidence of ARDS following amiodarone was 9.4% versus 0% in the placebo group.

Tisdale and colleagues[28,29] reported the results of two randomized studies of amiodarone prophylaxis for AF following general thoracic surgery that demonstrated effectiveness against AF without the increased risk of pulmonary toxicity suggested in the Van Mieghem and colleagues[24] study. The first report included 130 patients undergoing pulmonary resection, which concluded that amiodarone (at a dose of 1050 mg IV over 24 hours beginning at anesthesia induction and continuing at 400 mg orally twice a day until discharge or 6 days) reduced postoperative AF from 32.3% to 13.8% (P = .02). Approximately 25% of the patients in the study underwent pneumonectomy and there was no increase in the incidence of perioperative ARDS in the patients who received amiodarone prophylaxis.[28] Tisdale and colleagues[29] also reported the results of study of 80 esophagectomy patients who were randomized to amiodarone or no therapy. The amiodarone cohort received 4200 mg IV over 96 hours beginning during anesthesia induction. The incidence of postoperative AF requiring treatment was 15% versus 40% favoring amiodarone. The incidence of ARDS in the amiodarone cohort was 0%.

Given the results of the two studies from Tisdale and colleagues,[28,29] it seems likely that amiodarone is a safe prophylaxis therapy for postoperative AF following general thoracic surgical procedures when the lower dosing regimen is used. In the study by Van Mieghem and colleagues[24] that demonstrated a high incidence of ARDS after amiodarone therapy, higher dosing was used and an IV loading dose was given. Nevertheless, to err on the side of caution, given the availability of diltiazem, which is also effective, the authors believe that, until additional data are available, amiodarone prophylaxis should be avoided in patients with substantial preexisting pulmonary dysfunction or in those who may require pneumonectomy. For esophagectomy, amiodarone prophylaxis seems to be safe and at least as effective as diltiazem.[29]

BETA BLOCKER PROPHYLAXIS

In the general thoracic patient population, there are two randomized, double-blinded, controlled trials involving 129 participants that compared placebo to beta blockers in the prevention of postoperative AF.[30,31] In these two trials, beta blocker therapy (metoprolol and propranolol) did reduce postoperative AF from 23.1% to 9.4% (RR 0.40l; 95% CI, 0.17–0.95). Postoperative morbidity, however, was substantially higher in the beta blocker studies than in the studies involving calcium blockers. The incidence of hypotension was 49% with beta blockers, compared with 26% with placebo. In addition, bradycardia was 24.5% with beta blockers versus 4% with placebo. Pulmonary edema was also increased with an incidence of 14.1% for beta blockers compared with 6.2% in the placebo groups. Given the increased potential for hypotension and bradycardia, beta blockers appear to be a less viable choice for prophylaxis of AF. They should only be used in the setting of restarting beta blockers that a patient had already been taking preoperatively (to prevent beta blocker "withdrawal"), and they should be restarted at an initial dose that is approximately one-half of the preoperative dose to avoid potential side effects.

MAGNESIUM PROPHYLAXIS

Magnesium levels are often followed closely after general thoracic surgery procedures and maintained at between 1.8 mg/dL and 3.0 mg/dL. Lower serum magnesium level is independently associated with postoperative AF following cardiac surgery, and magnesium supplementation has been comprehensively studied in that population.[32] Shiga and colleagues[33] reported a meta-analysis of 17 trials in 2069 patients undergoing cardiac surgery and demonstrated a risk reduction for supraventricular arrhythmia of 23% with magnesium prophylaxis. There has been only one prospective, randomized trial evaluating magnesium prophylaxis in patients undergoing general thoracic surgery. Terzi and colleagues[34] reported on 194 patients undergoing lung resections and demonstrated a reduction in the incidence of AF to 10.7% from 26.7% (RR 0.40; 95% CI, 0.21–0.78; $P = .008$). The investigators did not report any cases of hypotension, bradycardia, and or severe pulmonary complications. The results of this study suggest that magnesium may be beneficial for AF prophylaxis in the general thoracic surgery patient population. At a minimum, magnesium levels should be maintained within the normal range.

Treatment of AF

There are times when, despite attempts at prophylaxis, optimal treatment of postoperative AF becomes essential. **Fig. 1** shows an algorithm for management of postoperative AF.

Postoperative AF in hemodynamically stable patients can be safely treated with rate-controlling agents alone because new-onset postoperative AF is often transient and self-limiting, and drugs used to control rate are generally safer than are those designed to achieve chemical cardioversion. Rena and colleagues[10] reported a study of 200 lung resection patients that demonstrated that 98% of postoperative AF resolved within 1 day of hospital discharge with rate-control alone. Approximately 50% of the episodes of postoperative AF spontaneously convert to normal sinus rhythm within 12 hours.[35]

The Atrial Fibrillation Follow-up Investigation of Rhythm Management (AFFIRM) trial was designed to examine whether an attempt at chemical conversion to normal sinus rhythm was beneficial compared with a rate-control strategy and anticoagulation in medical (non-postoperative) AF.[36] The AFFIRM trial enrolled 4060 patients who were randomized to rhythm control or rate control and followed for an average of 3.5 years. The rate-control group was treated with digoxin, beta

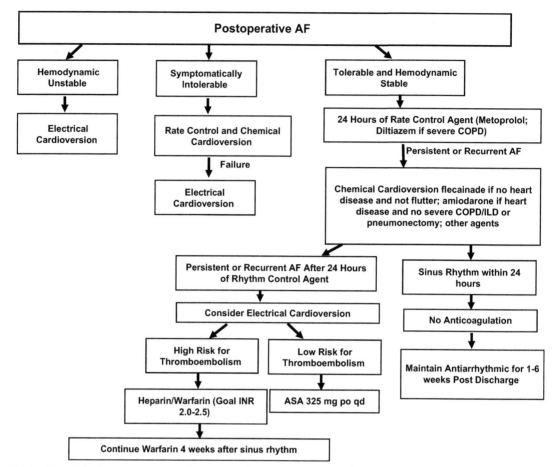

Fig. 1. Algorithm for management of postoperative AF. ILD, interstitial lung disease.

blockers and/or calcium channel blockers, and anticoagulation with warfarin (international normalized ratio [INR] 2.0–3.0). The rhythm control group was treated with antiarrhythmic drugs, including amiodarone, disopyramide, flecainide, moricizine, procainamide, and sotalol. Electrical cardioversion was also used as necessary to maintain normal sinus rhythm. The trial demonstrated no difference in the mortality rate and cerebral vascular accident rate between the rate-control strategy and rhythm-control strategy. The cost of the rate-control strategy was less. Although these results are not directly applicable to the postoperative AF population, they do make one wonder whether "knee-jerk" antiarrhythmic therapy in postoperative AF is indicated.

In patients who have persistent or recurrent AF after surgical procedures despite administration of rate-controlling agents, one must decide whether to continue with the rate-control strategy or attempt cardioversion to restore normal sinus rhythm. The reasons for restoration and maintenance of sinus rhythm in all (including medical AF)

patients include relief of symptoms, prevention of thromboembolism, and potentially avoidance of cardiomyopathy. In the surgical patient, however, issues surrounding the prevention of thromboembolism become paramount because of the increased risks of anticoagulation postoperatively.

Because most surgeons would like to avoid anticoagulation early postoperatively to minimize the chances of postoperative hemorrhage, a reasonable strategy for postoperative AF is to attempt cardioversion with antiarrhythmic medications before the need for anticoagulation arises. The support for this recommendation includes the many studies that demonstrate, in both postoperative and medical patients, that chemical cardioversion with antiarrhythmic agents are more likely to restore normal sinus rhythm in the short-term than is therapy with rate-control agents.[36–39] Because chemical cardioversion is likely to be effective within 24 hours, anticoagulation is avoided. On the other hand, the evidence of the usually transient nature of new-onset postoperative AF indicates that it might be reasonable for patients to simply be started on rate-control and anticoagulation therapy, when indicated, and then monitored closely for the resolution of AF in the outpatient setting. This approach would avoid the costs and side effects of antiarrhythmic therapy, but would incur anticoagulation in at least some patients.

When it is decided to attempt rate control for initial management of postoperative AF, the three classes of therapeutic agents available are beta blockers, calcium-channel blockers, and digoxin. Diltiazem has been proven to control ventricular rate more rapidly than digoxin following coronary bypass surgery.[40] Beta blocker therapy and calcium blocker therapy have demonstrated similar effectiveness in rate control in the medical AF population, and both classes of drugs are more effective than digitalis.[41] Because postoperative AF is considered partly related to an elevated adrenergic state, beta blockers may be a more preferable option, and they do seem to be more effective than calcium channel blockers in accelerating the conversion to sinus rhythm following noncardiac surgery.[42] In the nonsurgical population, metoprolol and atenolol generated improvement in both resting and exercise rate control.[43–45]

The potential concern with the use of beta blockers in COPD patients undergoing general thoracic surgery is the nonspecific beta-2 receptor blockade that may lead to bronchospasm. Although this occurs with some frequency with the use of nonspecific beta blockers such as propranolol, the data indicate that beta-1 specific agents, such as metoprolol, have a dramatically lower risk of inducing clinically significant bronchospasm.[46,47] Given the findings of these reports, the use of a selective beta-1 antagonist as the first-line rate-controlling agent in all patients except those with moderate or greater COPD would be an optimal strategy. Patients who are at greater risk for an exacerbation of bronchospasm (moderate-to-severe COPD patients) are more reasonably rate controlled with calcium channel blocker therapy.

The authors believe it is most reasonable to give rate-control agents alone a 24 hour trial to see if this will allow restoration of normal sinus rhythm. Beyond 24 hours, to reduce length of stay and minimize the rate of anticoagulation, it is reasonable to attempt chemical cardioversion with rhythm-control agents. Antiarrhythmic drugs that are designed to achieve chemical cardioversion are categorized into several classes and act by a variety of mechanisms. Antiarrhythmic agents studied in clinical trials include amiodarone, disopyramide, dofetilide, flecainide, ibutilide, procainamide, propafenone, quinidine, and sotalol. In AF that is not postoperative, randomized, controlled trials have demonstrated strong efficacy for acute cardioversion with amiodarone, dofetilide, flecainide, ibutilide, and propafenone; and moderate efficacy with quinidine.[48] A randomized study in cardiac surgery patients confirmed the better side-effects profile of amiodarone compared with quinidine.[49] Reisinger and colleagues[50] reported a prospective, randomized study of chemical cardioversion of AF after cardiac surgery that demonstrated equivalence of flecainide and ibutilide. Because of the higher rates of torsades des pointes with quinidine (up to 12%), the *American College of Cardiology/American Heart Association/European Society of Cardiology2006 Guidelines for the Management of Patients with Atrial Fibrillation*[51] does not recommend quinidine as a first-line agent. Patient characteristics that are specific to general thoracic surgical patients would make amiodarone and flecainide the more suitable antiarrhythmic agents. Many of the patients undergoing pulmonary resection have some degree of COPD; therefore, sotalol and propafenone would be less desirable choices given the risk of bronchospasm. Ibutilide and dofetilide are only available in IV forms and dofetilide is associated with torsades, which makes these agents less practical to use for treatment of postoperative AF.

The rates of chemical cardioversion that have been reported with amiodarone following general thoracic surgery range from 76% to 86%.[39,52] The conversion rates for flecainide are between 56% and 93%, but were found to be in the 80% range in most studies.[49,50,53] The major side effects of flecainide include atrial flutter, bradycardia, transient hypotension (IV form only), and mild neurologic side effects. Based the results of the Cardiac Arrhythmia Suppression Trial (CAST) Trial,[54] the major limitation on the use of flecainide is that it is strictly contraindicated in patients with any form of structural heart disease. In this trial, 323 patients were randomized to receive flecainide or encainide to suppress ventricular ectopy after myocardial infarction. The treatment groups had a worse outcome and a higher mortality rate because of arrhythmia or cardiogenic shock.

The side effects of amiodarone also include bradycardia and transient hypotension, and noncardiac, acute side effects can include phlebitis at the site of an IV infusion, hyperthyroidism or hypothyroidism, skin photosensitivity, hepatic dysfunction, neurologic changes (tremor, ataxia, and insomnia), and nausea and constipation with oral administration. In contrast to flecainide, amiodarone seems to be equally effective in AF and atrial flutter. The specific side effect of amiodarone, which has received the most attention and is highly pertinent to the general thoracic surgical population, is its pulmonary toxicity. The most commonly reported pulmonary toxic side effect is pulmonary fibrosis, which has been reported mainly in patients receiving large doses of the drug over prolonged periods of time, but it is clear that pulmonary toxicity also may occur less commonly in a fulminant form (interstitial pneumonitis) after even a short course of IV therapy. As mentioned above, a prospective, randomized trial of prophylactic amiodarone for patients undergoing lung surgery was stopped early because of the occurrence of ARDS at a far higher than expected rate (27%) in patients undergoing pneumonectomy.[24] Given the possibility of significant amiodarone-induced pulmonary toxicity in patients following pulmonary resection, flecainide or another agent for chemical cardioversion is indicated in patients who are mechanically ventilated, those with severe COPD, and following pneumonectomy.

Given the effectiveness and side-effect profiles of the various antiarrhythmic agents, amiodarone or flecainide seem to be the best choices for chemical cardioversion of AF after general thoracic surgery. Flecainide should not be used in patients with any form of structural heart disease. Amiodarone should be used with extreme caution in patients with significant baseline pulmonary dysfunction or who have undergone pneumonectomy, and IV doses should not exceed 1050 mg per day. In patients with both structural heart disease and substantial pulmonary dysfunction in whom chemical cardioversion is being considered, it is recommended to either initiate therapy with one of the other antiarrhythmic agents or attempt electrical cardioversion. The other alternative would be to initiate a rate-control strategy with calcium channel blockers or beta blockers in conjunction with anticoagulation.

Anticoagulation

Anticoagulation with warfarin has demonstrated efficacy for the prevention of stoke in several large, prospective clinical trials in nonsurgical patients with AF. However, the exact role of anticoagulation for postoperative AF after general thoracic operations has not been evaluated in clinical trials. As a result, there are limited data pertaining specifically to this setting and treatment recommendations must be extrapolated from the clinical trials of AF in nonsurgical patients. The clinical risk factors for the development of stroke in medical AF include previous stroke, transient ischemic attack, hypertension, age greater than 70 years, diabetes, congestive heart failure, and female gender.[5,55,56]

The primary therapeutic options for anticoagulation include warfarin and aspirin. Several

randomized trials have evaluated the efficacy of anticoagulation with these drugs.[57–60] A pooled analysis of these randomized clinical trials involved 3665 patients and demonstrated a reduction in yearly stroke rate from 4.5% to 1.4% in patients treated with warfarin. The overall RR reduction was 68%. Most of the strokes occurred in patients who had either discontinued warfarin therapy or had an INR level that was subtherapeutic.

Regarding aspirin, an analysis of pooled data from three randomized clinical trials identified a RR reduction of stroke with aspirin of 21% (95% CI, 0%–38%).[61] In a meta-analysis of 16 randomized trials, warfarin therapy decreased the RR of stroke by 62%, compared with aspirin, which only reduced the RR of stroke by 22%.[62] With regard to aspirin dosing, the Stroke Prevention in Atrial Fibrillation (SPAF) trial, which evaluated a dose of aspirin of 325 mg daily, resulted in the greatest reduction of the annual rate of stroke of any aspirin study by 42% compared with placebo (absolute reduction from 6.3% to 3.6%).[59]

The increased risk of bleeding associated with anticoagulation becomes more relevant in postoperative general thoracic surgery patients than in medical AF patients. Even in the medical patient, the risk of serious hemorrhage is greater with warfarin than with aspirin.[5] Hart and colleagues[63] conducted a meta-analysis of antithrombotic therapy to prevent stroke and found that warfarin increased the risk of major extracranial hemorrhage by 70% and intracranial hemorrhage by 128%.

Because most patients with postoperative AF will convert to sinus rhythm in the perioperative period, the time during which they are at risk for thromboembolism and stroke is narrow. In select situations, therefore, it may be reasonable to delay anticoagulation initially and institute warfarin therapy only if the patient remains in AF several days or weeks after the procedure. Further, the use of aspirin 325 mg daily rather than warfarin as the initial antithrombotic agent for AF would serve as a viable alternative for patients who do not display several of the risk factors for stoke (listed above) and may be at risk for postoperative bleeding at the surgical site. Specifically, the authors recommend that patients at a high risk for thromboembolism with a history stroke or transient ischemic attack, and patients with two or more risk factors for thromboembolism (heart failure, hypertension, diabetes, and age >75) receive anticoagulation therapy with warfarin. Patients without a history of stoke and patients with a single risk factor for thromboembolism can treated with aspirin 325 mg as an alternative to warfarin. Certainly, the risk of bleeding will be different between a patient who has undergone a video-assisted thoracoscopic surgery wedge resection compared with a patient who has undergone a transthoracic esophagectomy with extensive mediastinal and abdominal dissection. The extent of the surgery should be taken into consideration when deciding between warfarin and aspirin therapy in patients with persistent postoperative AF.

SUMMARY

AF commonly affects patients after general thoracic surgery. Postoperative AF increases hospital stay and charges. Effective prophylaxis and treatment is the goal. Calcium channel blockers prevent postoperative AF. Beta blockers are a less viable choice. Amiodarone prophylaxis should be avoided in patients with pulmonary dysfunction or who require pneumonectomy. When managing AF, a brief trial of rate-control agents is appropriate; however, chemical cardioversion with rhythm-control agents should be instituted after 24 hours. High-risk patients with history of stroke or transient ischemic attack or with two or more risk factors for thromboembolism should receive anticoagulation therapy.

REFERENCES

1. Vaporciyan AA, Correa AM, Rice DC, et al. Risk factors associated with atrial fibrillation after noncardiac thoracic surgery: analysis of 2588 patients. J Thorac Cardiovasc Surg 2004;127:779–86.
2. Bloom HL. Concise review of atrial fibrillation: treatment update considerations in light of AFFIRM and RACE. Clin Cardiol 2004;27:495–500.
3. Fernando HC, Jaklitsch MT, Walsh GL, et al. The society of thoracic surgeons practice guideline on the prophylaxis and management of atrial fibrillation associated with general thoracic surgery: executive summary. Ann Thorac Surg 2011;92(3):1144–52.
4. Falk RH. Etiology and complications of atrial: insights from pathology studies. Am J Cardiol 1998;821:10N–7N.
5. Falk RH. Atrial fibrillation. N Engl J Med 2001;344: 1067–78.
6. Konnings KT, Kirchof CJ, Smeets JR, et al. High-density mapping of electrically induced atrial fibrillation in humans. Circulation 1994;89:1665–80.
7. Cooklin M, Gold MR. Implications and treatment of atrial fibrillation after cardiothoracic surgery. Curr Opin Cardiol 1998;13:20–7.
8. Haïssaguerre M, Jaïs P, Shah DC, et al. Spontaneous initiation of atrial fibrillation by ectopic beats originating in the pulmonary veins. N Engl J Med 1998;339:659–66.
9. Asamura H, Naruke T, Tsuchiya R, et al. What are the risk factors for arrhythmias after thoracic operations? A retrospective multivariate analysis of 267 consecutive thoracic operations. J Thorac Cardiovasc Surg 1993;106:1104–10.
10. Rena O, Papalia E, Oliaro A, et al. Supraventricular arrhythmias after resection surgery of the lung. Eur J Cardiothorac Surg 2001;20:688–93.
11. Murthy SC, Law S, Whooley BP, et al. Atrial fibrillation after esophagectomy is a marker for postoperative morbidity and mortality. J Thorac Cardiovasc Surg 2003;126:1162–7.
12. Nielsen TD, Bahnson T, Davis RD, et al. Atrial fibrillation after pulmonary transplant. Chest 2004;126: 496–500.
13. Harpole DH, Liptay MJ, DeCamp MM, et al. Prospective analysis of pneumonectomy: risk factors for major morbidity and cardiac dysrythmias. Ann Thorac Surg 1996;61:977–82.
14. McKenna RJ Jr, Houck W, Fuller CB. Video-assisted thoracic surgery lobectomy: experience with 1,100 cases. Ann Thorac Surg 2006;81(2):421–5.
15. Paul S, Altorki NK, Sheng S, et al. Thoracoscopic lobectomy is associated with lower morbidity than open lobectomy: a propensity-matched analysis from the STS database. J Thorac Cardiovasc Surg 2010;139:366–78.
16. Onaitis MW, Petersen RP, Balderson SS, et al. Thoracoscopic lobectomy is safe and versatile procedure: experience with 500 consecutive patients. Ann Surg 2006;244:420–5.
17. Nattel S, Rango RE, Van Loon G. Mechanism of propranolol withdrawal phenomena. Circulation 1979;59:1158–64.
18. Salazar C, Frishman W, Friedman S, et al. Beta-Blockade therapy for supraventricular tachyarrhythmias after coronary surgery: a propranolol withdrawal syndrome? Angiology 1979;30:816–9.
19. Abel RM, Van Gelder HM, Pores IH, et al. Continued propranolol administration following coronary bypass surgery. Antiarrhythmic effects. Arch Surg 1983;118: 727–31.
20. Kalman JM, Munawar M, Howes LG, et al. Atrial fibrillation after coronary artery bypass grafting is associated with sympathetic activation. Ann Thorac Surg 1995;60:1709–15.
21. Sedrakyan A, Treasure T, Browne J, et al. Pharmacologic prophylaxis for postoperative atrial tachyarrhythmia in general thoracic surgery: evidence from randomized clinical trials. J Thorac Cardiovasc Surg 2005;129:997–1005.
22. Amar D, Roistracher N, Rusch VW, et al. Effects of Diltiazem prophylaxis on the incidence and clinical outcome of atrial arrhythmias after thoracic surgery. J Thorac Cardiovasc Surg 2000;120:790–8.

23. Lindgren L, Lepantalo M, von Knorring J, et al. Effect of Verapamil on right ventricular pressure and atrial tachyarrhythmia after thoracotomy. Br J Anaesth 1991;66:205–11.

24. Van Mieghem W, Coolen L, Malysse I, et al. Amiodarone and the development of ARDS after lung surgery. Chest 1994;105:1642–5.

25. Van Mieghem W, Tits G, Demuynck T, et al. Verapamil as prophylactic treatment for atrial fibrillation after lung operations. Ann Thorac Surg 1996;61:1083–5.

26. Amar D, Roisttracher N, Burt ME, et al. Effects of Diltiazem versus digoxin in dysrhythmias and cardiac function after pneumonectomy. Ann Thorac Surg 1997;63:1374–81.

27. Shimada M, Namai H, Morisaki H, et al. Preventative use of diltiazem to suppress supraventricular tachyarrhythmia in the patients after esophagectomy. Masui 1997;46:658–63.

28. Tisdale JE, Wroblewski HA, Wall DS, et al. A randomized trial evaluating amiodarone for prevention of atrial fibrillation after pulmonary resection. Ann Thorac Surg 2009;88:886–93.

29. Tisdale JE, Wroblewski HA, Wall DS, et al. A randomized, controlled study of amiodarone for prevention of atrial fibrillation after transthoracic esophagectomy. J Thorac Cardiovasc Surg 2010;140:45–51.

30. Jacobsen CJ, Bille S, Ahlburg P, et al. Perioperative metoprolol reduces the frequency of atrial fibrillation after thoracotomy for lung resection. J Cardiothorac Vasc Anesth 1997;11:746–51.

31. Bayliff CD, Massel DR, Inculet RI, et al. Propranolol for the prevention of postoperative arrhythmias in general thoracic surgery. Ann Thorac Surg 1999;67:182–6.

32. Casthely PA, Yoganathan T, Komer C, et al. Magnesium and arrhythmias after coronary artery bypass surgery. J Cardiothorac Vasc Anesth 1994;8:188–91.

33. Shiga T, Wajima Z, Inoue T, et al. Magnesium prophylaxis for arrhythmias after cardiac surgery: a meta-analysis of randomized controlled trials. Am J Med 2004;117:325–33.

34. Terzi A, Furlan G, Chiavacci P, et al. Prevention of atrial tachyarrhythmias after non-cardiac thoracic surgery by infusion of magnesium sulfate. Thorac Cardiovasc Surg 1996;44:300–3.

35. Amar D. Postoperative atrial fibrillation. Heart Dis 2002;4:117–23.

36. Wyse DG, Waldo AL, DiMarco JP, et al. A comparison of rate control and rhythm control in patients with atrial fibrillation. N Engl J Med 2002;347:1825–33.

37. VanderLugt JT, Mattioni T, Denker S, et al. Efficacy and safety of ibutilide fumarate for the conversion of atrial arrhythmias after cardiac surgery. Circulation 1999;100:329–75.

38. Hilleman DE, Spinler SA. Conversion of recent-onset atrial fibrillation with intravenous amiodarone: a meta-analysis of randomized controlled trials. Pharmacotherapy 2002;222:66–74.

39. Khan IA, Metha NJ, Gowda RM. Amiodarone for pharmacological cardioversion of recent-onset atrial fibrillation. Int J Cardiol 2003;89:239–48.

40. Tisdale JE, Padhi ID, Goldberg AD, et al. A randomized, double-blind comparison of intravenous diltiazem and digoxin for atrial fibrillation after coronary artery bypass surgery. Am Heart J 1998;135:739–47.

41. Olshansky B, Rosen feld LE, Warner AL, et al. The atrial fibrillation follow-up investigation of rhythm management (AFFIRM) study: approaches to control rate in atrial fibrillation. J Am Coll Cardiol 2004;43:1201–8.

42. Basler JR, Martinez EA, Winters BD, et al. Beta-adrenergic blockage accelerates conversion to postoperative supraventricular tachyarrhythmias. Anesthesiology 1998;89:1052–9.

43. Lewis RV, McMurray J, McDevitt DG. Effects of atenolol, verapamil, and xamoterol on heart rate and exercise tolerance in digitalised patients with chronic atrial fibrillation. J Cardiovasc Pharmacol 1989;131:1–6.

44. Farshi R, Kistner D, Sarma JS, et al. Ventricular rate control in chronic atrial fibrillation during daily activity and programmed exercise: a crossover open-label study for five drug regimens. J Am Coll Cardiol 1999;33:304–10.

45. Channner KS, James MA, MacConnell T, et al. Beta-adrenoceptor blockers in atrial fibrillation: the importance of partial agonist activity. Br J Clin Pharmacol 1994;37:53–7.

46. Ormiston TM, Salpeter SR. Beta-blocker use in patients with congestive heart failure and concomitant obstructive airway disease: moving from myth to evidence-based practice. Heart Fail Monit 2003;4:45–54.

47. Khosla S, Kunjummen B, Khaleel R, et al. Safety of therapeutic beta-blockade in patients with coexisting bronchospastic airway disease and coronary artery disease. Am J Ther 2003;10:48–50.

48. McNamara RL, Tamariz IJ, Segal JB, et al. Management of atrial fibrillation: review of the evidence for the role of pharmacologic therapy, electical cardioversion, and echocardiography. Ann Intern Med 2003;139:1018–33.

49. McAlister HF, Luke RA, Whitlock RM, et al. Intravenous amiodarone bolus versus oral quinidine for atrial flutter and fibrillation after cardiac operations. J Thorac Cardiovasc Surg 1990;99:911–8.

50. Reisinger J, Gatterer E, Lang W, et al. Flecainide versus ibutilide for immediate cardioversion of atrial fibrillation of recent onset. Eur Heart J 2004;25:1318–24.

51. Fuster V, Ryden LE, Cannom DS, et al. ACC/AHA/ESC 2006 guidelines for the management of patients with atrial fibrillation. Europace 2006;8:651–745.

52. Barbetakis N, Vassiliadis M. Is amiodarone a safe antiarrhythmic to use in supraventricular tachyarrhythmias after lung cancer surgery? BMC Surg 2004;4:7.

53. Bernard EO, Schmid ER, Scmidlin D, et al. Ibutilide versus amiodarone in atrial fibrillation: a double-blinded, randomized study. Crit Care Med 2003; 31:1031–4.

54. Echt DS, Liebson PR, Mitchell LB, et al. Mortality and morbidity in patients receiving encainide, flecainide, or placebo. The Cardiac Arrythmia Suppression Trial. N Engl J Med 1991;324:781–8.

55. Atiral Fibrillation Investigators. Risk factors for stroke and efficacy of antithrombotic therapy in atrial fibrillation. Analysis of pooled data from five randomized controlled trials. Arch Intern Med 1994;154:1449–57.

56. Hart RG, Pearce LA, McBride R, et al. Factors associated with ischemic stroke during aspirin therapy in atrial fibrillation: analysis of 2012 participants in the SPAF I–III clinical trials. The Stroke Prevention in Atrial Fibrillation (SPAF) Investigators. Stroke 1999; 30:1223–9.

57. Petersen P, Boysen G, Godtfredson J, et al. Placebo-controlled, randomised trial of warfarin and aspirin for prevention of thromboembolic complications on chronic atrial fibrillation. The Copenhagen AFASAK study. Lancet 1989;1:175–9.

58. The effect of low-dose warfarin on the risk of stroke in patients with nonrheumatic atrial fibrillation. The Boston Area Anticoagulation Trial for Atrial Fibrillation Investigators. N Engl J Med 1990;323: 1505–11.

59. Stroke Prevention in Atrial Fibrillation Investigtors. Stroke Prevention in Atrial Fibrillation study. Final results. Circulation 1991;84:527–39.

60. Ezekowitz MD, Bridges SL, James KE, et al. Warfarin in the prevention of stroke associated with nonrheumatic atrial fibrillation. Veterans Affairs Stroke Prevention in Nonrheumatic Atrial Fibrillation Investigators. N Engl J Med 1992;327:1406–12.

61. The efficacy of aspirin in patients with atrial fibrillation. Analysis of pooled data from 3 randomized trials. The Atrial Fibrillation Investigators. Arch Intern Med 1997;157(11):1237–40.

62. Hart RG, Benavente O, McBride R, et al. Antithrombotic therapy to prevent stroke in patients with atrial fibrillation: a meta-analysis. Ann Intern Med 1999; 131:492–501.

63. Hart RG, Pearce LA, Aguilar MI. Meta-analysis: antithrombotic therapy to prevent stroke in patients who have nonvalvular atrial fibrillation. Ann Intern Med 2007;146:857–67.

Deep Vein Thrombosis/ Pulmonary Embolism: Prophylaxis, Diagnosis, and Management

Alessandro Brunelli, MD

KEYWORDS

- Venous thromboembolism • Deep venous thrombosis
- Pulmonary embolism • Prophylaxis • Diagnosis • Therapy

Venous thromboembolism (VTE), which includes both deep vein thrombosis (DVT) and pulmonary embolism (PE), is a major cause of morbidity and mortality in hospitalized patients. It has been estimated that more than 450,000 patients are hospitalized annually in the United States for VTE.[1] Because only 1 in every 3 cases of VTE is detected, the actual number of cases in the United States may be about 1,350,000 annually. An analysis of data from the International Cooperative Pulmonary Embolism Registry revealed a crude 3-month mortality rate from VTE as high as 17.5%.[2] Venous thromboembolism has few specific symptoms and is clinically "silent" in most patients, making diagnosis difficult and unreliable. For this reason, prophylactic treatment methods are recommended for patients at risk for VTE.[3]

Thoracic surgery includes major interventions, which are increasingly performed in elderly and unfit patients with underlying cardiovascular and pulmonary comorbidities. As such, these patients must be considered at high risk for postoperative VTE.

DEEP VEIN THROMBOSIS

Specific guidelines are lacking for thoracic surgery. Hence recommendations must be extrapolated from more generic guidelines.

The most recent and widely accepted guidelines are those proposed by the National Institute for Health and Clinical Excellence (NICE)[4] and those from the American College of Chest Physicians (ACCP).[5]

Risk Factors and Risk Stratification

Both these guidelines[4,5] emphasize that VTE prophylaxis must be individualized according to the estimated risk of developing this complication.

The risk is estimated according to the type and extent of surgical procedure and to the presence of additional characteristics of patients.[5,6] A list of possible risk factors is summarized in **Box 1**.

The NICE guidelines[5] also recommend to assess all patients for risk of bleeding before offering pharmacologic VTE prophylaxis, and to not offer pharmacologic VTE prophylaxis to patients with the following risk factors for bleeding unless the risk of VTE outweighs the risk of bleeding: active bleeding, acquired bleeding disorders (ie, acute liver failure), concurrent use of anticoagulants (ie, warfarin with international normalized ratio >2), epidural or spinal anesthesia expected within the next 12 hours or performed within the previous 4 hours, acute stroke, thrombocytopenia, uncontrolled systolic hypertension (230 mm Hg or higher), and untreated inherited bleeding disorders (ie, hemophilia or von Willebrand disease).

VTE Prophylaxis: Summary of Guidelines

There are few data available in the literature regarding the risk and prevention of VTE in

The author has nothing to disclose.

Section Minimally Invasive Thoracic Surgery, Division of Thoracic Surgery, Ospedali Riuniti Ancona, Via Conca 1, Ancona 60122, Italy

E-mail address: brunellialex@gmail.com

Thorac Surg Clin 22 (2012) 25–28
doi:10.1016/j.thorsurg.2011.08.014

Box 1
Risk factors for venous thromboembolism

- Surgery (particularly if the expected total anesthetic and surgical time is longer than 90 minutes)
- Major trauma or injury of lower limbs
- Immobility
- Cancer
- Cancer therapy (hormonal, chemotherapy, angiogenesis inhibitors, radiotherapy)
- Active heart or respiratory failure
- Venous compression
- Previous VTE
- Age >60 years
- Dehydration
- Critical care admission
- Pregnancy and postpartum period
- Varicose veins with associated phlebitis
- Estrogen-containing oral contraceptives or hormone replacement therapy
- Selective estrogen receptor modulators
- Erythropoiesis-stimulating agents
- Acute medical illness
- Inflammatory bowel disease
- Nephrotic syndrome
- Myeloproliferative disorders
- Paroxysmal nocturnal hemoglobinuria
- Obesity (body mass index >30 kg/m^2)
- Central venous catheterization
- Inherited or acquired thrombophilia

Box 2
ACCP recommendations for VTE prophylaxis in thoracic surgery patients

1. For patients undergoing major thoracic surgery, a routine thromboprophylaxis with low molecular weight heparin (LMWH), low-dose unfractionated heparin (LDUH), or fondaparinux is recommended (grade of recommendations: strong recommendation, low or very low quality of evidence).

2. For thoracic surgery patients with a high risk of bleeding, the optimal use of mechanical thromboprophylaxis with properly fitted graduated compression stockings and/or intermittent pneumatic compression is recommended (grade of recommendations: strong recommendation, low or very low quality of evidence).

---

thoracic surgical centers. In the knowledge that the peak incidence of PE is 1 to 2 weeks after surgery, extending the prophylaxis even after discharge has become important. Many studies have shown that an extended prophylaxis reduced the incidence of DVT in patients submitted to major surgery for cancer.[7–9]

Therefore, an extended pharmacologic prophylaxis to 28 days postoperatively for patients who have had major cancer surgery is recommended.[10]

ACUTE PULMONARY EMBOLISM
Risk Stratification

The principal markers that are used to stratify the risk of acute PE may be grouped into 3 categories: clinical, of right ventricular (RV) dysfunction, and of myocardial injury.[11]

noncardiac thoracic surgery. Most of the available recommendations are therefore extrapolated from guidelines for major general surgical procedures.

The most commonly used published guidelines are those proposed by the ACCP and the NICE. **Box 2** shows recommendations proposed by the ACCP that are specific to thoracic surgery.[4]

Box 3 shows recommendations proposed by NICE guidelines that are specific to thoracic surgery.[5]

Duration of VTE Prophylaxis

In modern clinical practice an increasing number of patients leave the hospital sooner after the operation. A median stay of 4 to 6 days after major pulmonary resection is now the rule in many

---

Box 3
NICE guidelines specific to thoracic surgery

1. Start mechanical VTE prophylaxis at admission (choose any one of antiembolism stockings, foot impulse devices, intermittent pneumatic compression devices)

2. Continue mechanical VTE prophylaxis until the patient no longer has significantly reduced mobility

3. Add pharmacologic VTE prophylaxis (LMWH or unfractionated heparin) to patients who have a low risk of major bleeding, taking into account individual patient factors and according to clinical judgment

---

Clinical markers include the presence of shock or hypotension (defined as a systolic blood pressure <90 mm Hg or a pressure drop of >40 mm Hg for longer than 15 minutes if not caused by new-onset arrhythmia, hypovolemia, or sepsis).

Markers of RV dysfunction include evidence on echocardiography of RV dilatation, hypokinesis, or pressure overload; evidence on spiral computed tomography (CT) of RV dilatation; brain natriuretic peptide (BNP) or N-terminal pro-BNP elevation; elevated right heart pressure at right heart catheterization.

Markers of myocardial injury include the presence of a positive cardiac troponin T or I.

According to the combined presence of one or more of these markers, one can estimate the risk of PE-related early mortality.[11]

The concomitant presence of all risk markers is associated with a high risk of PE-related early mortality (>15%). In this circumstance thrombolysis or embolectomy is indicated.

If markers of RV dysfunction or myocardial injury, or both, are present, the PE-related mortality risk is about 3% to 15%. In this circumstance, home admission is recommended.

When none of the risk markers are present, the PE-related early mortality risk is low (<1%). Early discharge and home treatment may be indicated in this case.[11]

Diagnosis

The European Society of Cardiology has proposed diagnostic algorithms in cases of suspected high-risk and non–high-risk PE.[11]

In patients with suspected high-risk PE (ie, presenting with shock or hypotension), if the CT scan is not immediately available or if the critical conditions of the patient permit only bedside evaluation, echocardiography is particularly helpful in emergency management decisions. In a patient with shock or hypotension, the absence of echocardiographic signs of RV overload or dysfunction practically excludes PE as a cause of hemodynamic compromise. In this case, thrombolysis or embolectomy is not justified.[11] When CT scan is immediately available and the patient's conditions are stable, CT remains the test of choice. If the CT scan is positive, PE-specific treatment is justified.[11]

In patients with suspected non–high-risk PE (without shock or hypotension), CT angiography has become the main thoracic imaging test for investigating suspected PE. However, because most patients with suspected PE do not have the disease, CT should not be the first-line test. In patients admitted to the emergency department, plasma D-dimer measurement combined with clinical probability assessment is the logical first step and allows PE to be ruled out in around 30% of patients.[11] In the case of D-dimer measurement being positive or the clinical probability of PE being high, multidetector CT scanning should be performed.

Therapy

Hemodynamic and respiratory support is necessary in patients with suspected or confirmed PE presenting with shock or hypotension.

Anticoagulation with unfractionated heparin, LMWH, or fondaparinux should be initiated without delay in patients with confirmed PE and in those with a high or intermediate clinical probability of PE while the diagnostic workup is still ongoing. Except for patients at high risk for bleeding and those with severe renal dysfunction, subcutaneous LMWH or fondaparinux rather than intravenous unfractionated heparin should be considered for initial treatment.[11,12]

Several randomized controlled trials[13–18] have shown that thrombolytic therapy rapidly resolves thromboembolic obstruction and exerts beneficial effects on hemodynamic parameters.

For this reason, thrombolytic therapy should be regarded as the first-line treatment in patients with high-risk PE presenting with cardiogenic shock and/or persistent arterial hypotension.[11,12]

Conversely, routine use of thrombolysis in non–high-risk patients is not recommended, but may be considered in selected patients with intermediate-risk PE and after thorough consideration of conditions that increase the risk of bleeding (ie, hemorrhagic stroke, ischemic stroke in preceding 6 months, central nervous system damage or neoplasm, recent major trauma, surgery or head injury within preceding 3 weeks, gastrointestinal bleeding within the last month, known bleeding). Finally, thrombolytic therapy should not be used in patients with low-risk PE.[11,12]

For high-risk PE patients in whom thrombolysis is absolutely contraindicated or has failed, pulmonary embolectomy or, as an alternative, catheter embolectomy or fragmentation are valuable therapeutic options.[11,12]

SUMMARY

1. For patients undergoing major thoracic surgery without increased risk of bleeding, a routine thromboprophylaxis with LMWH heparin or LDUH, or fondaparinux is recommended. For

those patients at increased risk of bleeding, the optimal use of mechanical thromboprophylaxis is recommended. An extended pharmacologic prophylaxis to 28 days postoperatively for patients who have had major cancer surgery is recommended.

2. Anticoagulation with unfractionated heparin, LMWH, or fondaparinux should be initiated without delay in patients with confirmed PE and in those with a high or intermediate clinical probability of PE while the diagnostic workup is still ongoing. Thrombolytic therapy should be regarded as the first-line treatment in patients with high-risk PE presenting with cardiogenic shock and/or persistent arterial hypotension. Routine use of thrombolysis in non–high-risk patients is not recommended.

REFERENCES

1. Goldhaber SZ. Pulmonary embolism. Lancet 2004; 363:1295–305.

2. Goldhaber SZ, Visani L, De Rosa M. Acute pulmonary embolism: clinical outcomes in the International Cooperative Pulmonary Embolism Registry (ICOPER). Lancet 1999;353:1386–9.

3. Geerts WH, Heit JA, Clagett PG, et al. Prevention of venous thromboembolism. Chest 2001;119(Suppl 1): 132S–75S.

4. Reducing the risk of venous thromboembolism (deep vein thrombosis and pulmonary embolism) in patients admitted to hospital. National Institute for Health and Clinical Excellence; 2010. (NICE clinical guideline No. 92.) Available at: http://guidance.nice.org.uk/CG92. Accessed June 30, 2011.

5. Geerts WH, Bergqvist D, Pineo GF, et al. American College of Chest Physicians. Prevention of venous thromboembolism: American College of Chest Physicians Evidence-Based Clinical Practice Guidelines (8th edition). Chest 2008;133:381S–453S.

6. Anderson FA Jr, Spencer FA. Risk factors for venous thromboembolism. Circulation 2003;107:I9–16.

7. Lausen I, Jensen R, Jorgensen LN, et al. Incidence and prevention of deep venous thrombosis occurring late after general surgery: randomised controlled study of prolonged thromboprophylaxis. Eur J Surg 1998;164:657–63.

8. Bergqvist D, Agnelli G, Cohen AT, et al. Duration of prophylaxis against venous thromboembolism with enoxaparin after surgery for cancer. N Engl J Med 2002;346:975–80.

9. Rasmussen MS. Preventing thromboembolic complications in cancer patients after surgery: a role for prolonged thromboprophylaxis. Cancer Treat Rev 2002;28:141–4.

10. Treasure T, Chong LY, Sharpin CE. Perioperative prophylaxis against venous thromboembolism in major lung resection. In: Ferguson M, editor. Difficult decision in thoracic surgery. An evidence based approach. London: Springer-Verlag London Limited; 2011. p. 165–9.

11. Torbicki A, Perrier A, Konstantinides S, et al. ESC Committee for Practice Guidelines (CPG). Guidelines on the diagnosis and management of acute pulmonary embolism: the Task Force for the Diagnosis and Management of Acute Pulmonary Embolism of the European Society of Cardiology (ESC). Eur Heart J 2008;29:2276–315.

12. Jaff MR, McMurtry MS, Archer SL, et al. American Heart Association Council on Cardiopulmonary, Critical Care, Perioperative and Resuscitation; American Heart Association Council on Peripheral Vascular Disease; American Heart Association Council on Arteriosclerosis, Thrombosis and Vascular Biology. Management of massive and submassive pulmonary embolism, iliofemoral deep vein thrombosis, and chronic thromboembolic pulmonary hypertension: a scientific statement from the American Heart Association. Circulation 2011;123:1788–830.

13. Goldhaber SZ, Haire WD, Feldstein ML, et al. Alteplase versus heparin in acute pulmonary embolism: randomized trial assessing right-ventricular function and pulmonary perfusion. Lancet 1993;341:507–11.

14. Dalla-Volta S, Palla A, Santolicandro A, et al. PAIMS 2: alteplase combined with heparin versus heparin in the treatment of acute pulmonary embolism. Plasminogen Activator Italian Multicenter Study 2. J Am Coll Cardiol 1992;20:520–6.

15. Levine M, Hirsh J, Weitz J, et al. A randomized trial of a single bolus dosage regimen of recombinant tissue plasminogen activator in patients with acute pulmonary embolism. Chest 1990;98:1473–9.

16. Marini C, Di Ricco G, Rossi G, et al. Fibrinolytic effects of urokinase and heparin in acute pulmonary embolism: a randomized clinical trial. Respiration 1988;54:162–73.

17. Ly B, Arnesen H, Eie H, et al. A controlled clinical trial of streptokinase and heparin in the treatment of major pulmonary embolism. Acta Med Scand 1978;203:465–70.

18. Tibbutt DA, Chesterman CN. Pulmonary embolism: current therapeutic concepts. Drugs 1976;11:161–92.

The Management of Anticoagulants Perioperatively

Robert J. Cerfolio, MD*, Ayesha S. Bryant, MSPH, MD

KEYWORDS

- Thromboembolism • Anticoagulant • Warfarin
- Clopidogrel • Preoperative • Thoracic surgery

As obesity becomes more prevalent in society, as life expectancy climbs, and as the indications for the placement of stents in many vessels expand, the number of patients who are scheduled for thoracic surgery who are on anticoagulation or antiplatelet therapy continues to increase. In patients who are scheduled to undergo elective thoracic surgery, the surgeon must balance the need to optimize stent patency and yet minimize the patient's risk of thromboembolism (TE) and operative bleeding. Surgery itself increases the risk of TE by initiating a prothrombotic effect by increasing biochemical levels of clotting factors such as fibrinogen and D dimer.[1,2] Despite the evidence that surgery increases the risk of venous TE, there is currently no evidence that surgery itself increases the risk of arterial TE.[3]

The perioperative management of anticoagulants is influenced by several factors unique to each patient, which include (1) indication for the anticoagulation therapy initially (eg, atrial fibrillation, myocardial dysfunction, or prosthetic heart valve); (2) risk of hemorrhage (eg, the type of procedure to be performed); (3) patients' characteristics (eg, age, comorbidities, other drugs the patient is taking, weight) and their current international normalized ratio (INR), prothrombin time, partial thromboplastin time, and platelet count; (4) dose and type of anticoagulant being used and duration of anticoagulation; and (5) the operation to be performed. Like most issues in medicine,

each patient's care must be considered as a unique entity. **Boxes 1** and **2** attempt to objective this inherently subjective art. In this article, we address the perioperative management of the most commonly used anticoagulants seen in practice today, such as warfarin, heparin, dabigatran, clopidogrel, and aspirin, for the most commonly performed general thoracic operations.

WARFARIN

The American College of Chest Physicians (ACCP) proposed guidelines for antithrombotic prophylaxis in patients with different risk factors. The ACCP recommends that warfarin (Coumadin, Jantoven) therapy can be withheld for 4 to 5 days in patients who are at low risk for TE before the procedure without bridging.[4] In our practice, we have come to favor 5 days for mediastinoscopy and for minimally invasive esophageal and pulmonary surgery but 7 days for median sternotomy. In patients who are at moderate or high risk for TE, warfarin therapy should be stopped 5 days before the operation and then bridged using enoxaparin sodium (Lovenox; Sanofi-Aventis, Bridgewater, NJ, USA) or heparin. The decision to choose one or the other depends on the indications for warfarin initially and on the patient's risk factors for TE as shown in **Box 1**. For most elective thoracic operations (pulmonary resection either using minimally invasive techniques or open thoracotomy), the

Disclosures: Robert J. Cerfolio: ePlus Healthcare, speaker; Ethicon, speaker/consultant; NeoMend, consultant; OSI Pharmaceuticals, speaker; Atrium, consultant/speaker; Covidien, speaker; Precision, consultant/speaker; Intuitive, speaker. Ayesha Bryant: None.
Division of Cardiothoracic Surgery, University of Alabama at Birmingham, 703 19th Street South, ZRB 739, Birmingham, AL 35294, USA
* Corresponding author.
E-mail address: rcerfolio@uab.edu

Thorac Surg Clin 22 (2012) 29–34
doi:10.1016/j.thorsurg.2011.09.007

Box 1
Grading of patient risk for TE

High risk

Bridge with intravenous heparin or low-molecular-weight heparin

- Hypercoagulable state, history of TE, and 1 of the following:
  - Protein C or S deficiency, antithrombin III deficiency
  - Homozygous for clotting factor V Leiden mutation
  - Antiphospholipid antibody syndrome
- History of 2 or more arterial or idiopathic venous TE events
- TE within past 1 to 3 months
- Acute intracardiac thrombus shown by echocardiography
- Atrial fibrillation plus mechanical heart valve
- Older mechanical valve in mitral position
- Mechanical valve placed within 3 months
- Patients with bare metal stent placed within 6 weeks[a]
- Patients with drug-eluting stent within 12 months[a]

Intermediate risk

Bridging on patient-by-patient basis

- Cerebrovascular disease with 2 or more strokes/transient ischemic attack without risk factors for cardiac embolism
- Newer mechanical valve model in mitral position
- Older mechanical valve in aortic position
- Atrial fibrillation without history of cardiac embolism but with risks for cardiac embolism (eg, ejection fraction less than 40%, diabetes mellitus, hypertension, nonrheumatic valvular heart disease, transmural myocardial infarction within 1 month)
- Venous TE within the last 3 to 6 months

Low risk

No bridging or bridge with prophylactic or subtherapeutic dose of heparin

- One TE longer than 6 months ago
- Intrinsic cerebrovascular disease (carotid artery stenosis of more than 70%) without recurrent strokes/
- Atrial fibrillation without multiple risks for cardiac embolism
- Newer model prosthetic valves in aortic position

[a] Recommendation is to continue aspirin and clopidogrel.
  Data from Douketis JD, Berger PB, Dunn AS, et al. The perioperative management of antithrombotic therapy: American College of Chest Physicians Evidence-Based Clinical Practice Guidelines (8th edition). Chest 2008;133(Suppl 6): 299S-339S.

INR should be between 1.0 and 1.7, with a platelet count of 50,000 or more. Although much is made of the theoretical concern of rebound hypercoaguable states of abruptly stopping warfarin before surgery, this condition seems to occur rarely.[5]

THIENOPYRIDINES

Thienopyridines include clopidogrel (Sanofi-Aventis, Bridgewater, NJ, USA), ticlopidine (Ticlid;

Hoffmann-La Roche, Nutley, NJ, USA), and prasugrel.

Thienopyridines are platelet aggregation inhibitors that are often used in patients who have had previous cerebrovascular events or recent acute coronary events or are most commonly used in those who have had a coronary artery stent placed.[6] Recently, a surgical dictum that surgery was not safe in patients taking anticoagulants such as clopidogrel[7] was challenged by some general thoracic surgeons. Because of the increased risk of coronary thrombosis, the standard of care after the percutaneous insertion of a metal and/or drug-eluting stent is to place a patient on thienopyridines and aspirin. These agents reach their peak activity after 3 to 5 days and have a prolonged antiplatelet effect of 7 to 10 days. Several reports have shown the dramatic increased risk of coronary thrombosis of up to 29% if clopidogrel is withdrawn prematurely in patients with recently placed stents. In fact, a sudden withdrawal of clopidogrel has been shown to have a rebound effect with an increase in the hypercoagulation and prothrombotic state.[8–11] The recent recommendation from the American Heart Association's Science Advisory Committee is that patients who have undergone placement of a drug-eluting coronary artery stent should remain on dual antiplatelet therapy for at least12 months.[12]

These landmark recommendations changed the landscape of preoperative management of these patients all over the world. Many institutions held emergency meetings between the heads of cardiology, anesthesiology, and surgery. Hospitals and administrators scrambled to promulgate hospital policies for these patients. The result was a swirling morass of anxiety, chaos, and confusion. These rules mandated that no patients should have their clopidogrel stopped for 6 months if they had a sirolimus stent placed in their coronary arteries, for 3 months if they had a paclitaxel stent, or for 1 month if they had a bare metal stent. Thus, patients with known malignancies who underwent a preoperative stress test and failed and require a coronary stent often received a bare metal stent, followed by 1 month of clopidogrel and then surgery 1 or 2 weeks later. This decision led to the compromised therapy of not just 1 but 2 problems. It compromised the patient's coronary artery disease treatment with perhaps a nonoptimal stent and simultaneously delayed their cancer surgery for at least 6 weeks. In addition, it exposed these patients to a higher risk of perioperative myocardial infarction. Because of this complicated, volatile, and politically charged situation, we decided to assess the safety of a less-volatile and simpler solution: operating on patients who were taking clopidogrel.

Our article in 2010 was a prospective safety study consisting of 33 patients who continued clopidogrel in the perioperative period.[13] There were no statistically significant differences between the outcomes of these 33 patients who were taking clopidogrel up to and on the day of surgery and that of those who were not on anticoagulation therapy. Patients underwent a large variety of general thoracic operations, including lung resection (video-assisted thoracoscopic surgery or thoracotomy), esophagogastrectomy, mediastinoscopy, and sternotomy. Variables that were examined included operative time, hospital length of stay, estimated blood loss, or morbidity when stratified by procedure. In addition, we found that clopidogrel should be continued because it actually offered a protective effect against perioperative myocardial infarction, especially in those who have a coronary artery stent as their indication for antiplatelet therapy. However, we found an increased risk of bleeding secondary to the take down of adhesions in those patients who are to undergo a redo thoracotomy and who were taking both clopidogrel and aspirin. For these patients, we recommend that they stop their aspirin but continue their clopidogrel alone. By verbal report, we are aware that several other centers have adopted this regimen and their early initial results, although not yet published, are similar to ours. Thus it seems that performing surgery in patients taking clopidogrel is safe. Moreover, it may be the preferred management for those who are taking clopidogrel because of the deployment of a coronary artery stent deployment in the last 6 to 9 months, as opposed to stopping the medicine before general thoracic surgery.

HEPARIN

The half-life of unfractionated intravenous heparin is approximately 45 minutes.[14] Thus, it is often selected as a bridge to surgery in patients who have an absolute indication for anticoagulation, such as those with low-profile mechanical valves on the left side of the heart. Intravenous heparin should be stopped about 6 hours preoperatively.[4] Low-molecular-weight heparin also has a half-life of about 4 to 6 hours. Heparin is also commonly used as a bridge to surgery for patients on Coumadin and has the advantage that it can be given subcutaneously as opposed to heparin that is given intravenously. Most guidelines suggest that the last dose of subcutaneous low-molecular-weight heparin should be given 24 to 48 hours preoperatively.

DABIGATRAN

Dabigatran is an oral reversible direct thrombin inhibitor that is sometimes used in patients who have renal impairment for the prevention of venous thromboemboli. It has a predictable pharmacokinetic profile, and thus frequent routine blood work monitoring coagulation is often not needed unlike in Coumadin. Dabigatran's peak anticoagulant activity is 2 to 3 hours after ingestion, and it has a half-life of 12 to 14 hours in patients with normal renal function (and approximately 28–30 hours in those with severe renal impairment).[15,16] Dabigatran should be discontinued 1 to 2 days preoperatively in patients with a creatinine clearance of 50 mL/min or more. For those patients with renal impairment (creatinine clearance <50 mL/min), it should be discontinued 3 to 5 days before the procedure. If the patient requires conversion to a parenteral anticoagulant, it is best to wait for 12 (creatinine clearance ≥30 mL/min) to 24 hours (creatinine clearance <30 mL/min) after the last dose of dabigatran before initiating the parenteral anticoagulant.[16,17]

OTHER ANTICOAGULANTS

Aspirin irreversibly inhibits platelet cyclooxygenase. It has a half-life of 15 to 20 minutes; however, because it irreversibly binds platelets, its effect persists the duration of the platelet's life span, which is approximately 7 to 10 days.[18] When aspirin is stopped for 4 to 5 days, approximately 50% of platelets return to normal function, and thus many patients are instructed to stop their aspirin only for

this duration before surgery by their internists, as opposed to 7 to 10 days. Recent studies show that stopping aspirin therapy for 5 or more days in patients with underlying cardiovascular disease may increase the risk of acute coronary syndrome or stroke.[19] The 2008 ACCP guidelines recommend that patients who are at high risk for thromboemboli in whom there is no high risk of hemorrhage for the planned operation should continue aspirin in the perioperative period. If aspirin is discontinued preoperatively, it should be resumed approximately 24 hours (or the following morning) after surgery depending on the patient's clinical status.[4]

DIPYRIDAMOLE

Dipyridamole (Persantine) is a combination vasodilator and antiplatelet agent. Its half-life is approximately 10 hours. It is more frequently used in patients with a past medical history of a cerebrovascular event.[20] At present, there are no set guidelines on the perioperative management of patients who are using dipyridamole; however, we recommend stopping it for 4 to 5 days in patients who are to undergo elective procedure if their risk of repeat stroke is low and the operation is at most a pulmonary or esophageal resection.

The cessation of anticoagulants before general thoracic surgery is variable and depends as much on the patient's risk factors as it does on the type of operation that is to be performed. We are more liberal with the use of anticoagulants if we are to perform a lobectomy via a thoracotomy than via a robotic approach. Similarly, we are even more conservative when performing a video mediastinoscopy in which vessels and/or bleeding tissues are not ligated or stapled but rather can only be cauterized or compressed. These factors must be taken into account, and the risks and benefits must be decided for each patient by each surgeon. The decision as to when to restart anticoagulants after surgery must also be based on each individual's risks.

RESUMPTION OF ANTICOAGULANTS POSTOPERATIVELY

In general, the decision regarding the safe restart of anticoagulants after surgery is based on the patient's individual risks, the operation performed, and their clinical status after surgery. All recommendations in this article are for a patient who is not bleeding and is doing well clinically with no major complications. Obviously, if a patient is bleeding or has to be moved back to the operating room to treat some type of postoperative complication, then restarting anticoagulants is ill advised.

Warfarin

Warfarin should be restarted as soon as possible after the general thoracic surgical procedure. In most cases, it is usually restarted within 24 hours postoperatively, provided hemostasis is ensured.[4] However, the interval also depends on factors such as the number of chest tubes that are in the pleural space, the intraoperative blood loss, and the patient's individual risk factors for TE. If the patient is at low risk for TE, then warfarin can be restarted, even as early as postoperative day 2, after all the chest tubes have been removed. If an epidural has been placed, it should be removed before restarting warfarin. If the patient is at high risk for TE, then it is prudent to attempt to remove the chest tubes sooner (at first ensuring there is no bleeding or chylothorax). If possible, we prefer to avoid an epidural in patients who were on warfarin preoperatively and who will need it restarted postoperatively.

Clopidogrel

Because we recommend not stopping clopidogrel, the question as to when best to restart it is moot. However, if it has been stopped before surgery (as it might be in a patient with a remote history of stroke without identified causes who not infrequently comes to a thoracic surgeon regarding it or for a redo operation), then it is reasonable to restart it in this type of low-risk patients after the chest tubes have been removed in the early postoperative period.

Heparin

Usually when heparin has been used preoperatively, it is because the patient is at high risk for TE, and thus early restarting is often desired. The onset of anticoagulation in patients using heparin is about 1 hour after administration, with peak anticoagulation levels at 3 to 5 hours. Given these parameters, heparin can usually be reinitiated safely 24 hours after the operation is over. However, delayed bleeding can occur and both the character and the amount of chest tube drainage needs to be carefully assessed before restarting heparin, especially in the high-risk operations shown in **Box 2**.

Dabigatran

Dabigatran therapy should be restarted when hemostasis has been achieved because its onset of action is rapid (2–3 hours). If heparin was used to bridge anticoagulant, dabigatran should be initiated less than 2 hours before the next scheduled dose of a parenteral anticoagulant or at the time intravenous anticoagulation is discontinued.[4]

The risk and benefits of stopping it and restarting it must be assessed for each patient.

Aspirin and Dipyridamole

Usually aspirin and dipyridamole can be restarted within 1 or 2 days after a general thoracic surgical procedure. The risk of bleeding when restarting these agents is low, and thus there should be little resistance to restarting them even with chest tubes still in place.

SUMMARY

Although there is little level 1 evidence from prospective randomized trials for the perioperative management of anticoagulants in patients who undergo general thoracic surgical operations, the recommendations in this article can be extrapolated from other literature. These guidelines have been implemented safely by many institutions. Communication between the thoracic surgeon, cardiologist, internal medicine physician, and anesthesiologist; a patient-by-patient consideration of the indication for anticoagulant therapy preoperatively; and the type of operation performed are paramount to minimizing the incidence of postoperative TEs events and bleeding complications.

REFERENCES

1. Rowbotham BJ, Whitaker AN, Harrison J, et al. Measurement of crosslinked fibrin derivatives in patients undergoing abdominal surgery: use in the diagnosis of postoperative venous thrombosis. Blood Coagul Fibrinolysis 1992;3(1):25.
2. Lip GY, Lowe GD. Fibrin D-dimer: a useful clinical marker of thrombogenesis? Clin Sci (Lond) 1995; 89:205.
3. Carter CJ. The pathophysiology of venous thrombosis. Prog Cardiovasc Dis 1994;36(6):439.
4. Douketis JD, Berger PB, Dunn AS, et al. The perioperative management of antithrombotic therapy: American College of Chest Physicians Evidence-Based Clinical Practice Guidelines (8th edition). Chest 2008;133(Suppl 6):299S–339S.
5. Palareti G, Legnani C, Guazzaloca G, et al. Activation of blood coagulation after abrupt or stepwise withdrawal of oral anticoagulants—a prospective study. Thromb Haemost 1994;72(2):222.
6. Weitz HI, Hirsh J, Samama MM. New antithrombotic drugs. Chest 2008;133:234S–56S.
7. Berger P, Verheugt F. Perioperative cardiac care: how to handle the clopidogrel. Pittsburgh: ACCEL; 2008.
8. Iakovou I, Schmidt T, Bonizzoni E, et al. Incidence, predictors, and outcome of thrombosis after successful implantation of drug-eluting stents. JAMA 2005; 293:2126–30.

9. Spertus JA, Kettelkamp R, Vance C, et al. Prevalence, predictors, and outcomes of premature discontinuation of thienopyridine therapy after drug-eluting stent placement: results from the PREMIER registry. Circulation 2006;113:2803–9.

10. Eisenstein EL, Anstrom KJ, Kong DF, et al. Clopidogrel use and long-term clinical outcomes after drug-eluting stent implantation. JAMA 2007;297:159–68.

11. Newsome LT, Weller RS, Gerancher JC, et al. Coronary artery stents. II: perioperative considerations and management. Anesth Analg 2008;107:570–90.

12. Grines CL, Bonow RO, Casey DE Jr, et al. Prevention of premature discontinuation of dual antiplatelet therapy in patients with coronary artery stents: a science advisory from the American Heart Association, American College of Cardiology, Society for Cardiovascular Angiography and Interventions, American College of Surgeons, and American Dental Association, with representation from the American College of Physicians. Circulation 2007; 115:813–8.

13. Cerfolio RJ, Minnich DJ, Bryant AS. General thoracic surgery is safe in patients taking clopidogrel. J Thorac Cardiovasc Surg 2010;140:970–6.

14. Hirsh J, Bauer KA, Donati MB, et al. American College of Chest Physicians. Parenteral anticoagulants: American College of Chest Physicians Evidence-Based Clinical Practice Guidelines (8th edition). Chest 2008;133(Suppl 6):141S.

15. Stangier J, Rathgen K, Stähle H, et al. Influence of renal impairment on the pharmacokinetics and pharmacodynamics of oral dabigatran etexilate: an open-label, parallel-group, single-centre study. Clin Pharmacokinet 2010;49(4):259.

16. Hankey GJ, Eikelboom JW. Dabigatran etexilate: a new oral thrombin inhibitor. Circulation 2011; 123(13):1436.

17. Van Ryn J, Stangier J, Haertter S, et al. Dabigatran etexilate—a novel, reversible, oral direct thrombin inhibitor: interpretation of coagulation assays and reversal of anticoagulant activity. Thromb Haemost 2010;103(6):1116.

18. Roth GJ, Majerus PW. The mechanism of the effect of aspirin on human platelets: I. Acetylation of a particulate fraction protein. J Clin Invest 1975;56: 624–32.

19. Ferrari E, Benhamou M, Cerboni P, et al. Coronary syndromes following aspirin withdrawal: a special risk for late stent thrombosis. J Am Coll Cardiol 2005;45(3):456.

20. Diener HC, Cunha L, Forbes C, et al. European Stroke Prevention Study. 2. Dipyridamole and acetylsalicylic acid in the secondary prevention of stroke. J Neurol Sci 1996;143(1-2):1.

Perioperative Antibiotics in Thoracic Surgery

Stephanie H. Chang, MD, Alexander S. Krupnick, MD*

KEYWORDS

- Perioperative antibiotics • General thoracic surgery
- Postoperative infection • Transplantation

Successful patient outcomes and low perioperative complications depend not only on surgical technique but pre and postoperative patient management as well. Antibiotic prophylaxis has rapidly advanced over the last several decades decreasing the morbidity of general thoracic procedures. While, unlike the case for abdominal or cardiac surgery, few randomized clinical trials have focused on the optimal antibiotic prophylaxis in general thoracic surgery evidence based practice guidelines do exist in the published literature to guide our practice.

DEFINITION OF SURGICAL SITE INFECTION

In 1992, the Surgical Wound Infection Task Force redefined surgical infections as surgical site infections (SSIs), involving infection of the incision or organs/spaces manipulated during an operative intervention.[1] Remote infections, not including bloodstream infections related to an SSI, are not included in the definition of SSI.[1] This task force split the categorization of SSIs into superficial incisional, deep incisional, and organ/space SSI (**Table 1**). SSIs need to manifest within 30 days of the operation, unless an implant was involved, in which case the time frame for deep incisional and organ/space SSIs is increased to 1 year. Superficial SSIs are confined to the skin and subcutaneous tissue, deep incisional SSIs involve deeper soft tissues, such as fascial planes and muscle layers, and organ/space SSIs include any anatomic location, excluding incisional area, that was manipulated during an operation. An exception to these SSI classifications occurs when an organ/space infection communicates with the skin and drains along the incision site, as this is considered an incisional complication, and defined as a deep incisional SSI. Of note, the strict definition of an SSI does not include "remote" postoperative infections, such as pneumonia after a nonthoracic surgery or a urinary tract infection after a nonurologic procedure.

HISTORY OF SURGICAL ANTIBIOTIC PROPHYLAXIS

After the development of anesthetic techniques in the mid-nineteenth century, the surgeon was poised to expand the range and complexity of operative procedures that could safely be performed; however, the complications resulting from infection related to such intervention led to continued difficulty with postoperative morbidity and mortality and severely limited the scope of disease processes that could be treated surgically. The work on antiseptic principles at the end of the nineteenth century was pivotal with regard to SSI control and modern-day antibiotic prophylaxis. Ignaz Semmelweis was the first to realize the impact of handwashing on postoperative complications, noting that puerperal fever was threefold higher in patients treated by physicians who participated in autopsies of patients who died from the same cause. Based on this finding, he mandated that physicians wash their hands in chlorine before patient interaction, decreasing mortality from 9.0% to 1.5%.[2] Louis

The authors have nothing to disclose.

Division of Cardiothoracic Surgery, Washington University in St Louis School of Medicine, 660 South Euclid, Campus Box 8234, St Louis, MO 63110-1013, USA

* Corresponding author.

E-mail address: krupnicka@wudosis.wustl.edu

Thorac Surg Clin 22 (2012) 35–45

doi:10.1016/j.thorsurg.2011.08.012

Table 1
Surgical site infections

	Tissue Involved	Time Frame	Symptoms
Incisional SSI			
Superficial	Skin and subcutaneous tissue	Within 30 days of surgery	One of: • Purulent discharge • Organism cultured from fluid or tissue • Pain, tenderness, swelling, erythema AND opened by surgeon • Diagnosis by surgeon or attending physician
Deep	Deep soft tissue (eg, fascial plane, muscles)	Within 30 days of surgery OR 1 year with implant	One of: • Purulent discharge • Spontaneous dehiscence OR opened by surgeon with fever or pain • Evidence on direct examination or radiology • Diagnosis by surgeon or attending physician
Organ/Space SSI[a]			
	Any anatomy manipulated during surgery other than incision	Within 30 days of surgery OR 1 year with implant	One of: • Purulent discharge from organ space • Organism cultured from fluid or tissue • Evidence on direct examination or radiology • Diagnosis by surgeon or attending physician

Abbreviation: SSI, surgical site infection.
[a] Note: If an organ/space infection communicates with the skin and drains along the incision, this is considered a deep incisional SSI.

Pasteur later demonstrated that infectious diseases are attributable to microbes, and developed techniques for sterilization. His work laid the groundwork for Joseph Lister, the father of antisepsis, who in 1867 used carbolic acid to dress wounds and decrease the incidence of infection and perioperative mortality. Other notable scientists, such as Robert Koch and William Osler, contributed to SSI treatment through techniques to isolate the infectious organisms. Their work led to the understanding that the host inflammatory response to infection can also lead to morbidity. All of these advances helped in understanding antisepsis and the role of microbial organisms in infection, paving the road to the discovery of prophylactic antibiotics.[3]

In 1928, Sir Alexander Fleming discovered the first effective antimicrobial. He left a Petri dish of bacteria uncovered during vacation, and on his return, he noted that Staphylococcus did not grow in or around a mold colony. Realizing the potential of this mold, he discovered penicillin. Following this, multiple other antibiotics were developed, and used for prophylaxis during operative intervention in the 1950s. The clinical trials at that time demonstrated no difference with antibiotic use, but their study design included multiple flaws, including lack of randomization, inappropriate antibiotic use, and inappropriate timing of prophylaxis. More recent randomized controlled trials have shown perioperative antibiotics to be advantageous for prevention of SSIs (**Table 2**).[4–7]

PRACTICE PATTERNS OF SURGICAL PROPHYLAXIS IN THORACIC SURGERY
Evidence-Based Indications for Prophylaxis for Lung Resection

Efficacy of perioperative antibiotics
There have been multiple prospective randomized control trials regarding perioperative antibiotics for noncardiac thoracic surgery, but unfortunately

Table 2
Pivotal randomized control trials for perioperative antibiotic use

Trial, Year	Surgical Field	Antibiotic Regimen	Antibiotic Group Infection Rate	Control Group Infection Rate	P Value
Bernard and Cole,[4] 1964	Gastrointestinal surgery	Penicillin G/Methicillin/ Chloramphenicol vs placebo (given pre-, intra-, and postoperatively)	8% (5/66 patients)	27% (21/79 patients)	<.005
Brown et al,[5] 1969	Gastrointestinal, head and neck, hernia, skin, and soft tissue surgery	Cephaloridine vs placebo (given preoperatively then every 8 hours for 5–10 doses)	6.7% (6/90 patients)	22.8% (21/92 patients)	<.01
Allen et al,[6] 1972	Gynecologic procedures	Cephalothin vs placebo (given pre-, intra-, and postoperatively for 5 days)	14.1% (12/85 patients)	41.0% (34/83 patients)	<.001
Boyd et al,[7] 1973	Hip fractures	Nafcillin vs placebo (given pre-, intra-, and postoperatively)	0.8% (1/135 patients)	4.8% (7/145 patients)	.041

unlike the case for cardiac surgery,[8] no official guidelines exist. One of the earliest studies was performed was in 1977 by Kvale and colleagues.[9] It was a randomized, prospective double-blind study in patients undergoing pulmonary surgery, comparing cefazolin 500 mg intramuscularly (IM), starting on arrival to the operating room, followed by cefazolin 500 mg IM every 6 hours, then oral cephalexin 500 mg when the patient was tolerating a diet for a total of 5 days versus placebo treatment. The results of this study showed a statistically significant difference in perioperative infection with a 50% infection rate (17 of 34 patients) in the control group versus 19% in the perioperative antibiotic group (8 of 43 patients). This pivotal trial initiated the now common practice of using perioperative cephalosporin prophylaxis in thoracic surgery.

The subsequent 2 randomized trials, however, contradicted the findings of Kvale and colleagues,[9] creating confusion and putting into doubt the role of antibiotic prophylaxis in pulmonary resection. Truesdale and colleagues[10] treated patients with cephaloxin 1 g IM in the operating room before pulmonary resection, followed by 2 g intravenously (IV) every 6 hours for a total 48 hours or a placebo dosed in a similar fashion. Their data demonstrated a 17.2% (5 of 29 patients) infection rate in those receiving a placebo and a 17.8% (5 of 28 patients) rate of postoperative infection in those receiving antibiotics. A similar trial performed at the Johns Hopkins Medical Center[11] also did not demonstrate a difference in the rate of perioperative wound infection between patients receiving 2 g IV cephalothin versus placebo before and

6 hours after pulmonary surgery. They reported no statistical difference, but did not give a number for the wound infections.

Following these 2 trials, all subsequent studies reported an advantage to using perioperative antibiotics, swaying the clinicians toward antibiotic prophylaxis. In Toronto, Ilves and colleagues[12] randomized patients with esophageal or pulmonary surgery to cephalothin 2 g IV in the operating room followed by 2 g IV 4 hours later versus placebo. The results showed 23.7% (22 of 93) patients had wound infections in the placebo group, compared with 5.9% (7 of 118 patients) in the treatment group. They also demonstrated a non–statistically significant decrease in the postoperative pneumonia and empyema with prophylactic antibiotics. In 1982, Frimodt-Møller and colleagues[13] compared penicillin G 5 million international units (IU) IV before surgery and every 6 hours for a total of 5 doses versus placebo. Placebo resulted in a 19.1% (9 of 47 patients) wound infection rate, whereas the use of prophylactic antibiotics led to a 4.4% (2 of 45 patients) infection rate. Aznar and colleagues[14] revisited this topic in 1991. They designed another prospective, randomized, double-blind trial comparing cefazolin 1 g IV 30 minutes before surgery versus placebo. This trial, performed more than a decade after the previous 5 studies, supported the data in Kvale and colleagues',[9] Ilves and colleagues',[12] and Frimodt-Møller and colleagues'[13] trials, with a statistically significant decrease in wound infection from 14% (8 of 57 patients) in the placebo group versus 1.5% (1 of 70 patients) with perioperative antibiotics.

Additionally there was a decrease in empyema (14% vs 7%) and pneumonia (9% vs 4%) in the treatment arm. Thus, despite the small number of randomized clinical trials and initial conflicting data, most trials support the use of perioperative antibiotics in noncardiac thoracic surgery with a decrease in surgical site infection postoperatively. No consistent data, however, are available to demonstrate an effect of perioperative antibiotics on the rate of postoperative pneumonia or empyema.

Duration of perioperative antibiotics

Multiple studies have shown the efficacy of single-dose prophylactic antibiotics in other surgical procedures,[15–18] but few such trials have been conducted for pulmonary surgery. Olak and colleagues[19] performed the first prospective study looking at the appropriate course of perioperative antibiotics in 1991. Patients were randomized to cefazolin 1 g IV before induction of anesthesia or cefazolin 1 g IV at induction and every 8 hours for a total of 6 doses. This study showed no difference in SSIs, including wound infection, pneumonia, or empyema between the 2 arms. Subsequently, Wertzel and colleagues[20] randomized patients undergoing pulmonary resection to ampicillin/sulbactam 3 g at induction only versus 3 g at induction and every 8 hours for a total of 3 doses. Again, no difference was present between the single-dose and multidose antibiotic regimens. Other studies, including Aznar and colleagues,[14] looked at single-dose perioperative antibiotics versus placebo, and showed a significant decrease in SSIs, supporting the efficacy of single-dose antibiotics for pulmonary surgery.

One randomized controlled study, conducted by Bernard and colleagues[21] in 1994, supported the longer use of perioperative antibiotics, randomizing patients to cefuroxime 1.5 g IV before surgery and 2 hours later versus the same regimen plus doses every 6 hours postoperatively for 48 hours. Their data showed no change in superficial wound infections, but demonstrated a decreased incidence in empyema, from 15.6% with 2 doses down to 6.0% in the 48-hour treatment. These data are skewed, however, as 7 patients in the 2-dose group developed bronchopleural fistulas, compared with 2 patients in the 48-hour group, with broncho-pleural fistula most likely related to surgical technique. It is thus likely that the fistula was the cause for the increased incidence of infection in the 2-dose group, decreasing the validity of this study's findings.

Although a limited number of randomized controlled trials have investigated the appropriate duration of perioperative antibiotics for pulmonary surgery, based on these data we can conclude that a single dose of antibiotics before incision is effective at decreasing the incidence of SSIs. This conclusion is supported by the expansive number of trials in cardiac surgery that also demonstrate the efficacy of perioperative antibiotics, with a single dose of antibiotics as effective as up to 48 hours of prophylaxis.[8]

Selection of perioperative antibiotics

The choice of prophylactic antibiotics is based on the most common pathogens likely to result in SSI, which heavily depends on the operative procedure.[22] In pulmonary surgery, bacteria from normal skin and respiratory flora are the common cause of SSIs. These consist of Staphylococcus aureus, coagulase-negative staphylococci, Streptococcus pneumoniae, and gram-negative bacilli,[23,24] with S aureus being the most commonly identified pathogen. Cephalosporins provide adequate coverage over these organisms and are a good class of antibiotics for infection prophylaxis in pulmonary surgery. Although cephalosporins differ in their spectrum of coverage based on generation (first-generation through fourth-generation cephalosporins are currently available with increased coverage of gram-negative bacteria with increasing generation of drug), clinical trials have been unable to demonstrate a difference with regard to surgical site infection.[25,26]

Only one randomized controlled trial compared the use of first-generation versus third-generation cephalosporins, and was designed to elucidate the effect of third-generation cephalosporins' increased activity against gram-negative bacilli on perioperative complications. Turna and colleagues[26] randomized patients to a first-generation cephalosporin (cephalexin 1.5 g IV) before surgery, then every 12 hours, versus a third-generation cephalosporin (cefepime 1 g IV) before surgery, then every 24 hours, for a total of 48 hours for each group. Their results indicated no difference in SSIs postoperatively between the 2 groups, supporting the usage of first-generation cephalosporins given their decreased cost and better coverage against gram-positive organisms. This lack of difference between the cephalosporin classes is supported by multiple trials regarding SSI prevention in cardiac surgery.[25]

Summary

Therefore, first-generation cephalosporins, such as cefazolin, which have good coverage for the most common pulmonary SSIs, are an appropriate choice for prophylactic antibiotic therapy. The appropriate dosage for cefazolin is 1 to 2 g IV before incision.[27] If the patient has a history of methicillin-resistant *S aureus* or a penicillin allergy, than vancomycin 1 g IV can be used in place of cefazolin.

Evidence-Based Indications for Prophylaxis for Esophageal Surgery

Efficacy of perioperative antibiotics

The use of perioperative antibiotics in esophageal and gastroduodenal procedures is based on multiple randomized controlled trials, all of which overwhelmingly demonstrate a benefit from the use of perioperative antibiotic regimens. Because esophageal resections commonly involve gastroduodenal manipulation for conduit formation, our field relies significantly on data acquired by general surgeons for antibiotics in gastric surgeries to determine appropriate prophylaxis of esophageal surgery. Stone and colleagues[22] conducted one of the first large randomized controlled trials in 1976. They enrolled 400 patients undergoing elective gastric, biliary, and colonic surgery, and randomized them to 4 groups with cefazolin 1 g IV given as follows: (1) 8 to 12 hours before surgery, (2) 1 hour before surgery, (3) 1 to 4 hours postoperatively, or (4) never. The gastric arm had 96 patients, with a 5% (1 of 22 patients) superficial SSI rate 8 to 12 hours before surgery, 4% (1 of 27 patients) 1 hour before surgery, 17% (4 of 24 patients) 1 to 4 hours postoperatively, and 22%

(5 of 23 patients) if no antibiotics were given. These data demonstrate the efficacy of perioperative antibiotics, and the necessity of giving the antibiotics before incision. Additionally, there was a decrease in organ/space SSIs, as demonstrated by a decrease from a 9% rate of peritoneal sepsis in the no-treatment group to 4% in the groups treated 8 to 12 hours and 1 hour preoperatively.

Subsequent studies, such as that of Lewis and colleagues[28] in 1982 and Nichols and colleagues,[29] confirm the role of antimicrobial prophylaxis in decreasing SSIs. Lewis and colleagues[28] randomized patients to receiving perioperative cefamandole versus placebo in elective and emergent gastric procedures, and noted a decrease in the infection rate from 28% (8 of 28 patients) to 3% (1 of 32 patients). Nichols and colleagues[29] also randomized patients to cefamandole versus placebo for high-risk, elective gastroduodenal procedures. The placebo group had a 35% (7 of 20 patients) rate of infection compared with 5% (1 of 19 patients) in the treatment arm.

Rotman and colleagues[30] held a large randomized controlled trial that investigated the use of preoperative cefazolin or cefotaxime 1 g every 8 hours for 3 doses versus placebo for abdominal operations, enrolling more than 3000 patients. They studied the effect of perioperative antibiotics on clean, clean-contaminated, and contaminated resections (**Table 3**),[31,32] as well as on patients

Table 3
Surgical wound classification

	Definition[31]	Wound Infection Rate[32]
Clean	• No inflammation • No break in sterile technique • Genitourinary or biliary tract can be entered if no infected urine or bile • Gastrointestinal or respiratory tract are not entered • Transection of appendix or cystic duct without acute infection is considered clean	2.1%
Clean-Contaminated	• Minor break in sterile technique • Genitourinary or biliary tract entered with infected urine or bile • Gastrointestinal or respiratory tract entered without gross spillage	3.3%
Contaminated	• Major break in sterile technique (eg, cardiac massage) • Acute inflammation without presence of pus • Gastrointestinal tract gross spillage • Traumatic wound, fresh from relatively clean source	6.4%
Dirty	• Pus • Perforated viscus • Traumatic wound, old or dirty source	7.1%

with risk factors that predispose them to wound infections, such as diabetes, steroid use, and ascites. There was a statistically significant decreased incidence in infection across all groups between placebo and cefazolin, with a global reduction in postoperative wound abscesses from 5% to 2%. Cefotaxime had rates comparable to cefazolin. A decrease was noted in all 4 groups, with a decrease from 4% to 1% in patients with clean-contaminated operations and a 9% to 5% reduction in high-risk patients, again supporting the use of antimicrobials before abdominal surgery.[30]

Because of the strong evidence provided by randomized clinical trials, perioperative antibiotic therapy with esophageal, gastric, and duodenal surgeries are indicated to decrease the incidence of SSIs.

Duration of perioperative antibiotics
Many studies have focused on the duration of antibiotics for abdominal surgery, with some specific to gastric surgery. In 1976, Stone and colleagues[33] published a randomized trial of 220 patients undergoing gastric, biliary, and colonic surgery to cefamandole 1 g IM 1 hour before surgery, 1 g IV intraoperatively, and 1 g IV in the recovery room, followed by either placebo or cefamandole 1 g IM every 6 hours for 5 days. The gastric surgery arm demonstrated a 0% infection rate in the 25 patients with a short-course antibiotic regimen and the 29 patients with the 5-day antibiotic regimen, demonstrating no indication for prolonged perioperative antibiotics. They further evaluated this by looking at patients undergoing emergent laparotomy for abdominal trauma resulting in peritoneal contamination, and again demonstrated that there was no gain in prolonged antibiotic therapy for both superficial site infections (8% and 10%, respectively) and deep/organ space infections (4% vs 5%, respectively).[33]

These findings were corroborated when Lewis and colleagues[34] in 1991 studied the efficacy of a single perioperative antibiotic dose of intravenous cefotaxime versus a short postoperative course. Both groups demonstrated no incidence of superficial SSIs but a 3% incidence of a subphrenic abscess after anastamotic leak in both the single-dose and short antibiotic course (1 of 26 patients and 1 of 27 patients, respectively), supporting the use of a single dose of antibiotics.

Based on these randomized trials, and others looking at the efficacy of single-dose prophylaxis for abdominal surgery,[15–18] we conclude that a short course of perioperative antibiotics, and perhaps even a single dose of preoperative antibiotics, is successful at decreasing the occurrence of

SSIs associated with esophageal and gastroduodenal surgery. Thus, as described in **Table 4**, based on the best available data, antibiotic prophylaxis for general thoracic surgery in our institution, both pulmonary and esophageal, includes only a short course of perioperative antibiotics.

Selection of perioperative antibiotics
The most common pathogens present in SSIs for esophageal, gastric, and duodenal resection are enteric gram-negative bacilli, streptococci, and oropharyngeal anaerobes.[16,22,24,35,36] Given this spectrum of pathogens, cephalosporins again are an adequate class of antimicrobials for prophylaxis of postoperative infections. Most studies have evaluated first-generation, second-generation, and third-generation cephalosporins as perioperative antibiotics for gastroduodenal resection. The 1979 study by Stone and colleagues[33] also compared short-course cefamandole, a second-generation cephalosporin, to cephaloridine, a first-generation cephalosporin, with no significant difference in wound infections for gastric surgeries. The studies by Lewis and colleagues[28] and Nichols and colleagues[29] both demonstrated that cefamandole was effective at significantly decreasing SSIs in high-risk patients. The study by Rotman and colleagues[30] showed no significant difference between patients treated with cefazolin versus cefotaxime, with cefazolin having the statistically significant decrease in overall infection when compared with placebo. Therefore, no differences have been shown between each generation of cephalosporins on changing SSI rate for upper gastrointestinal surgeries.

The use of cefazolin, which has good coverage against gram-positive cocci and enteric gram-negative organisms, as a prophylactic antibiotic for esophageal, gastric, and duodenal resections is the most efficacious in light of a low anaerobic burden. The appropriate dosage is 1 to 2 g IV before incision,[27] and vancomycin 1 g IV if the patient has a history of methicillin-resistant *S aureus* or a penicillin allergy. For patients with a high anaerobic burden, such as may occur after esophageal perforation or Boerhaave syndrome, the use of a fourth-generation cephalosporin such as cefepime, which has greater anaerobic coverage, would likely prove to be more efficacious, although no current study has evaluated this hypothesis.

Evidence-Based Indications for Lung Transplantation

Perioperative antibiotic prophylaxis after lung transplantation is extremely important, as infection and bronchiolitis are the major causes of death in the first 5 years after transplantation.[37] This high

Table 4
Perioperative antimicrobial recommendations for thoracic surgery

	Common Pathogens	Antibiotic Regimen
Pulmonary resections	• Staphylococcus aureus • Coagulase-negative staphylococci • Streptococcus pneumoniae • Gram-negative bacilli	• Cefazolin 1 g IV preoperatively, with a total of 1–3 doses every 8 hours • If penicillin allergic, vancomycin 1 g IV preoperatively, with a total of 1–3 doses every 12 hours
Esophageal surgeries	• Enteric gram-negative bacilli • Streptococci • Oropharyngeal anaerobes	• Cefazolin 1 g IV preoperatively, with a total of 1–3 doses every 8 hours • If penicillin allergic, vancomycin 1 g IV preoperatively, with a total of 1–3 doses every 12 hours • If high anaerobic burden likely, cefepime 1 g IV preoperatively, with a total of 1–3 doses every 12 hours
Lung transplantation	• Pseudomonas • B Cepacia • Gram-negative bacilli • Methicillin-resistant Staphylococcus aureus • Cytomegalovirus • Candida • Aspergillosis • Pneumocystis carinii	• Cefepime 1 g IV preoperatively, with a 7–10-day course (based on the empiric experience of Washington University in St Louis) • For cystic fibrosis patients, sensitivities are sent and for multidrug-resistant Pseudomonas, inhaled colistin should be added perioperatively • Vancomycin 1 g IV preoperatively, with a 7–10-day course (based on the empiric experience of Washington University in St Louis) • For seropositive recipients, valganciclovir 900 mg PO daily or ganciclovir 5 mg IV 5 times per week while CMV PCR positive (based on the empiric experience of Washington University in St Louis) • For seronegative recipients with seropositive donors, valcyte 900 mg PO daily for 6 months (based on the empiric experience of Washington University in St Louis) OR ganciclovir 5 mg IV 5 times per week or 1 g PO TID for 6 months • Amphotericin B, itraconazole, or voriconazole for 1 year • Trimethoprim-sulfamethoxazole prophylaxis 3 times per week • For sulfa allergies, dapsone and inhaled pentamadine can be used

Empyema	• S aureus
	• Streptococcus milleri
	• Escherichia coli
	• Pseudomonas
	• Haemophilus influenzae
	• Klebsiella
	• Anaerobes
		Antibiotics should be based on culture and sensitivity from empyema. If not available, the following regimens are appropriate for 3 weeks
		• Community acquired (all are acceptable periop abx)
		  ○ Cefuroxime 500 mg IV TID + metronidazole 500 mg PO or 400 mg IV TID
		  ○ Penicillin 1 g QID + metronidazole 500 mg PO or 400 mg IV TID
		  ○ Meropenem 1 g TID + metronidazole 500 mg PO or 400 mg IV TID
		  ○ Augmentin 875/125 mg PO TID
		  ○ Amoxicillin 1 g PO TID + metronidazole 400 mg PO TID
		  ○ Clindamycin 300 mg PO QID
		• Hospital acquired (all are acceptable periop abx)
		  ○ Piperacillin-tazobactam 4.5 g IV QID
		  ○ Ceftazidime 2 g IV TID
		  ○ Meropenem 1 g IV TID ± metronidazole 500 mg IV TID or 400 mg PO TID

Abbreviations: abx, antibiotics; CMV, cytomegalovirus; IV, intravenous; PCR, polymerase chain reaction; periop, perioperative; PO, orally; preop, preoperative; QID, 4 times per day; TID, 3 times per day.

rate of infectious complications is a result of many factors, including immunosuppression, decreased mucociliary action, and continuous exposure to the outside environment and pathogens[38]; however, no standardized regimens or guidelines exist regarding the choice of perioperative antibiotic or antifungal therapy.[38,39]

Bacterial infections are the most common after transplantation, and pathogens are usually gram-negative rods, such as *Pseudomonas* and *Burkholderia cepacia*.[38] Thus, an antipseudomonal antibiotic with gram-negative bacilli coverage, such as cefepime, is appropriate for perioperative prophylaxis. *Staphylococcus* infections are also common postoperatively. Given the increased risk of methicillin-resistant *S aureus*, vancomycin is also routinely used in conjunction with a cephalosporin. These antibiotics are given for 7 to 10 days after transplantation and then discontinued unless the patient has a clinical indication for continued antibiotic therapy.[40,41] The routine use of trimethoprim-sulfamethoxazole (TMP-SMX) for *Pneumocystis carinii*, described later, is also adequate prophylaxis against development of rare bacterial infections, such as *Legionella, Listeria*, and *Nocardia*.[38]

Viral infections, most notably with cytomegalovirus (CMV), are the second most frequent source of infection in lung transplantation. CMV infections generally occur in the first 4 months after transplantation, and are most common in seronegative recipients (ie, those who have never been infected with the virus and thus have not developed protective antibodies) who receive CMV-positive lungs, or in patients who are seropositive but require increased immunosuppression to prevent rejection.[42] Common antiviral agents used in the postoperative period are ganciclovir, acyclovir, and valganciclovir. One randomized trial compared the efficacy of acyclovir to ganciclovir in prevention of CMV, using ganciclovir for the first 3 weeks, then either acyclovir 800 mg 4 times a day or ganciclovir 5 mg 5 times a week. At 90 days, the rate of CMV shedding or pneumonitis was 50% with acyclovir versus 15% with ganciclovir. Additionally, the acyclovir group had a greater rate (54%) of obliterative bronchiolitis, as a sequelae of CMV infection, compared with ganciclovir (17%).[43] Thus, ganciclovir is the preferred method of viral prophylaxis, compared with acyclovir. The efficacy of valganciclovir versus ganciclovir in patients with lung transplantation has not been extensively studied. No prophylaxis is indicated for seronegative donors and recipients. For seropositive recipients, with seropositive or seronegative donors, CMV polymerase chain reaction can be monitored, and prophylaxis can

be instituted if the infection is detected. Many institutions also choose to have universal prophylaxis in this subset of patients. With seronegative recipients and seropositive donors, prophylaxis is instituted with either IV ganciclovir or oral valganciclovir. Other viral infections, such as herpes simplex, also used to be prevalent, but since the routine use of antivirals in the postoperative period, their incidence has rapidly decreased.[44]

Fungal infections are less common than bacterial infections, accounting for 10% to 14% of infections after transplantation, but have a much higher mortality compared with bacterial infections.[38] The most common fungal pathogens are *Candida* and *Aspergillosis*, which generally occur within the first months after transplantation.[38] Most *Candida* species and *Aspergillosis* are sensitive to fluconazole, but the more resistant strains require treatment with amphotericin B.[45–47] In 1997, Reichenspurner and colleagues[47] published a thorough retrospective review demonstrating that amphotericin B significantly decreased the rate of invasive fungal infections after transplantation, from 20% to 8%. Later, Minari and colleagues[48] performed a similar retrospective review of their patients, focusing on itraconazole prophylaxis versus no prophylaxis, and found that 4.9% (4 of 81 patients) in the treated group developed aspergillosis, compared with 18.2% (16 of 88 patients) without treatment. Voriconazole has also been compared with fluconazole and itraconazole, with a decreased incidence of invasive aspergillosis, but increased hepatotoxicity and other side effects.[49] No other studies have directly compared amphotericin B versus the azoles, so no conclusions can be drawn except that all decrease the rate of postoperative fungal infections. *P carinii* is also a fungal infection that presents in the first 6 months after transplantation and occurred in up to 70% of patients before prophylactic regimens.[40] Current prophylaxis involves TMP-SMX, which has significantly decreased the incidence of *P carinii* infection. If patients cannot tolerate TMP-SMX, then dapsone and aerosolized pentamadine are appropriate alternatives.[38]

Special consideration applies to patients with cystic fibrosis undergoing lung transplantation. Because of prolonged exposure to antibiotics, they have increased proclivity to multidrug-resistant *Pseudomonas*. It has been shown that inhaled aminoglycosides, specifically inhaled colistin or tobramycin, decrease pseudomonal colonization.[50,51] Additionally, use of aerosolized colistin in patients with cystic fibrosis promotes an increase in pseudomonal sensitivity from multidrug-resistant *Pseudomonas*.[52] Thus, inhaled colistin, in addition to cefepime, is now routinely used in patients with cystic fibrosis whose pulmonary isolates demonstrate drug-resistant *Pseudomonas*. This has directly led to an increase in survival from lung transplantation.

Overall, there is a generalized lack of randomized trials regarding appropriate perioperative antimicrobial therapy for lung transplantation; however, because many retrospective studies have evaluated infections that occur after transplantation and the specific pathogens involved, a generalized guideline for antimicrobial use in lung transplantation can be established. Given the prevalence of gram-negative bacilli and methicillin-resistant *S aureus* infections, we routinely use perioperative cefepime and vancomycin in patients who receive transplants for nonsuppurative diseases. In those with cystic fibrosis, inhaled colistin should be added. Ganciclovir should be used for CMV prophylaxis, whereas amphotericin B, itraconazole, or voriconazole can be used for prevention of *Candida* and aspergillosis. TMP-SMX is routinely used for prevention of *P carinii*.

Evidence-Based Indications for Empyema

Empyema, or infection of the pleural space, is a sequelae of pneumonia and subsequential parapneumonic effusion that develops into frank pus.[53] Frequently these are managed by drainage with thoracostomy tubes or surgical drainage, in addition to perioperative antibiotics.[35] Gram-positive aerobes are the most common organisms, including *S aureus* and *Streptococcus milleri*.[54] Additionally, gram-negative aerobes, such as *Escherichia coli*, *Pseudomonas*, *Haemophilus influenzae*, and *Klebsiella*, are common, and occasionally occur in the presence of anaerobic organisms in empyemas.[54,55] Anaerobes can be the sole isolate from empyemas in roughly 14% of cases, with a greater insidious onset.[53] Most of these organisms are resistant to penicillin, but beta-lactams are appropriate for pseudomonal and *S milleri* infections. Both penicillin and cephalosporins penetrate the pleural space, whereas aminoglycosides do not and may not be effective for empyemas.[56,57] For community-acquired infections, *Pneumococcus*, *S aureus,* and *H influenzae* are the most common organisms, and a cephalosporin as well as a beta-lactamase inhibitor or metronidazole are appropriate owing to frequent penicillin-resistant aerobes and anaerobes.[53,58] Clindamycin alone will also adequately cover these common organisms.[58] Hospital-acquired empyemas are generally caused by nosocomial infections or trauma, so antibiotics should cover gram-positive and gram-negative aerobes and anaerobes, such as with piperacillin-tazobactam, meropenem, or third-generation cephalosporins.[53,56] There is no current recommended duration of antibiotic therapy, as the mainstay for the treatment of the infected pleural space is surgical drainage, but prolonged antibiotic treatment for roughly 3 weeks is appropriate based on clinical experience.[53] For possible appropriate perioperative antibiotic regimens, see **Table 4**.

SUMMARY

No official guidelines exist for perioperative antibiotic use in noncardiac thoracic surgery. Despite the original conflicting data and few randomized trials for prophylaxis in pulmonary resections, there is strong evidence supporting the use of a perioperative antibiotic, specifically cefazolin 1 to 2 g IV, before incision, then every 8 hours for a total of 1 to 3 doses. Regarding esophageal resection, strong data exist supporting the use of cefazolin, 1 to 2 g IV, before incision and then every 8 hours for a total of 1 to 3 doses. Despite lack of trials, however, we also suggest changing the antibiotic to cefepime 1 g IV before incision, then every 12 hours for 1 to 3 doses in patients who are at risk for high anaerobic burden (because of perforation, for example), as cefepime has better anaerobic coverage. If patients have a history of methicillin-resistant *S aureus* or a penicillin allergy, vancomycin 1 g IV should be substituted for cefazolin preoperatively and every 12 hours for a total of 1 to 3 doses. In lung transplant recipients who are at high risk for gram-negative bacilli (specifically pseudomonal), methicillin-resistant *S aureus*, CMV, *Candida,* aspergillosis, and *P carinii*, prophylaxis with cefepime, vancomycin, ganciclovir, antifungals, and TMP-SMX is warranted. Antifungal therapy can consist of amphotericin B, itraconazole, or voriconazole. If patients are allergic to sulfa, dapsone and inhaled pentamadine can be substituted. Patients with cystic fibrosis require extra prophylaxis with inhaled colistin because of their increased colonization with multidrug-resistant *Pseudomonas*. Perioperative antibiotic treatment for empyema should be based on cultures and sensitivities; however, if those are not available, multiple IV and oral options exist for management of community-acquired and hospital-acquired pneumonia with subsequential empyema (see **Table 4**).

REFERENCES

1. Horan TC, Gaynes TP, Martone WJ, et al. CDC definitions of nosocomial surgical site infections, 1992: a modification of CDC definitions of surgical

wound infections. Infect Control Hosp Epidemiol 1992;13(10):606–8.

2. Beilman GJ, Dunn DL, et al. Surgical infections. In: Brunicardi FC, Andersen DK, Billiar TR, et al, editors. Schwartz's principles of surgery. 9th edition. New York: McGraw-Hill Professional; 2009. Chapter 6.

3. Burke JF. The effective period of preventive antibiotic action in experimental incision and dermal lesions. Surgery 1961;50:161–8.

4. Bernard HR, Cole WR. The prophylaxis of surgical infection: the effect of prophylactic antimicrobial drugs on the incidence of infection following potentially contaminated operations. Surgery 1964;56: 151–9.

5. Brown JW, Cooper N, Rambo WM. Controlled prospective double-blind evaluation of a "prophylactic" antibiotic (cephaloridine) in surgery. Antimicrob Agents Chemother 1969;9:421–3.

6. Allen JL, Rampone JF, Wheeless CR. Use of a prophylactic antibiotic in elective major gynecologic operations. Obstet Gynecol 1972;39: 218–24.

7. Boyd RJ, Burke JF, Colton T. A double-blind clinical trial of prophylactic antibiotics in hip fractures. J Bone Joint Surg Am 1973;55:1251–8.

8. Edwards FH, Engelman RM, Houck P, et al. The society of thoracic surgeons practice guideline series: antibiotic prophylaxis in cardiac surgery, part I: duration. Ann Thorac Surg 2006;81:397–404.

9. Kvale P, Ranga V, Kopacz M, et al. Pulmonary resection. South Med J 1977;70:64–9.

10. Truesdale R, D'Alessandri R, Manuel V, et al. Antimicrobial vs placebo prophylaxis in noncardiac thoracic surgery. JAMA 1979;241:1254–6.

11. Cameron J, Imbembo A, Keiffer R, et al. Prospective clinical trial of antibiotics for pulmonary resection. Surg Gynecol Obstet 1981;152:156–8.

12. Ilves R, Cooper J, Todd T, et al. Prospective, randomized, double-blind study using prophylactic cephalothin for major, elective, general thoracic operations. J Thorac Cardiovasc Surg 1981;81: 813–7.

13. Frimodt-Møller N, Ostri P, Pedersen I, et al. Antibiotic prophylaxis in pulmonary surgery: a double- blind study of penicillin versus placebo. Ann Surg 1982; 195:444–50.

14. Aznar R, Mateu M, Miro J, et al. Antibiotic prophylaxis in non-cardiac thoracic surgery: cefazolin versus placebo. Eur J Cardiothorac Surg 1991;5: 515–8.

15. American Society of Health-System Pharmacists Commission on Therapeutics. ASHP therapeutic guidelines on antimicrobial prophylaxis in surgery. Am J Health Syst Pharm 1999;56:1839–88.

16. Mangram AJ, Horan TC, Pearson ML, et al. Guideline for prevention of surgical site infection, 1999. Hospital Infection Control Practices Advisory Committee. Infect Control Hosp Epidemiol 1999;20: 247–80.

17. DiPiro JT, Cheung RP, Bowden TA, et al. Single dose systemic antibiotic prophylaxis of surgical wound infections. Am J Surg 1986;152:552–9.

18. McDonald M, Grabsch E, Marshall C, et al. Single versus multiple-dose antimicrobial prophylaxis for major surgery: a systematic review. Aust N Z J Surg 1998;68:388–96.

19. Olak J, Jeyasingham K, Forrester-Wood C, et al. Randomized trial of one-dose versus six-dose cefazolin prophylaxis in elective general thoracic surgery. Ann Thorac Surg 1991;51:956–8.

20. Wertzel H, Swoboda L, Joos-Wurtemberger A, et al. Perioperative antibiotic prophylaxis in general thoracic surgery. Thorac Cardiovasc Surg 1992;40: 326–9.

21. Bernard A, Pillett M, Goudet P, et al. Antibiotic prophylaxis in pulmonary surgery: a prospective randomized double-blind trial of flash cefuroxime versus forty-eight-hour cefuroxime. J Thorac Cardiovasc Surg 1994;107:896–900.

22. Stone HH, Hooper CA, Kolb LD, et al. Antibiotic prophylaxis in gastric, biliary and colonic surgery. Ann Surg 1976;184:443–52.

23. Nichols RL, Smith JW, Muzik AC, et al. Preventative antibiotic usage in traumatic thoracic injuries requiring closed tube thoracostomy. Chest 1994; 106:1493–8.

24. Antimicrobial prophylaxis in surgery. Med Lett Drugs Ther 1999;41:75–80.

25. Engelman R, Shahian D, Shemin R, et al. The society of thoracic surgeons practice guideline series: antibiotic prophylaxis in cardiac surgery, part II: antibiotic choice. Ann Thorac Surg 2007;83:1569–76.

26. Turna A, Kutlu C, Ozalp T, et al. Antibiotic prophylaxis in elective thoracic surgery: cefuroxime versus cefepime. Thorac Cardiovasc Surg 2003;51:84–8.

27. Classen DC, Evans RS, Pestotnik SL, et al. The timing of prophylactic administration of antibiotics and the risk of surgical-wound infection. N Engl J Med 1992;326:281–6.

28. Lewis RT, Allan CM, Goodall RG, et al. Cefamandole in gastroduodenal surgery: a controlled, prospective, randomized, double-blind study. Can J Surg 1982;25:561–3.

29. Nichols TL, Webb WR, Jones JW, et al. Efficacy of antibiotic prophylaxis in high risk gastroduodenal operations. Am J Surg 1982;143:94–8.

30. Rotman N, Hay JM, Lacaine F, et al. Prophylactic antibiotherapy in abdominal surgery. First- vs third-generation cephalosporins. Arch Surg 1989;124: 323–7.

31. Howard JM, Barker WF, Culbertson WR, et al. Postoperative wound infections: the influence of ultraviolet irradiation of the operating room and of various other factors. Ann Surg 1964;160:1–192.

32. Culver DH, Horan TC, Gaynes RP, et al. Surgical wound infection rates by wound class, operative procedure, and patient risk index. National Nosocomial Infections Surveillance System. Am J Med 1991;91:152S–7S.

33. Stone HH, Haney BB, Kolb LD, et al. Prophylactic and preventive antibiotic therapy: timing, duration and economics. Ann Surg 1979;189:691–9.

34. Lewis RT, Goodall RG, Marien B, et al. Efficacy and distribution of single-dose preoperative antibiotic prophylaxis in high-risk gastroduodenal surgery. Can J Surg 1991;34:117–22.

35. Gatehouse D, Dimock F, Burdon DW, et al. Prediction of wound sepsis following gastric operations. Br J Surg 1978;65:551–4.

36. Lewis RT, Allan CM, Goodall RG, et al. Discriminate use of antibiotic prophylaxis in gastroduodenal surgery. Am J Surg 1979;138(5):640–3.

37. Hosenpud JD, Bennett LE, Keck BM, et al. The registry of the International Society for Heart and Lung Transplantation: sixteenth official report – 1999. J Heart Lung Transplant 1999;18:611–26.

38. Alexander BD, Tapson VF. Infectious complications of lung transplantation. Transpl Infect Dis 2001; 3(3):128–37.

39. Husain S, Zaldonis D, Kusne S, et al. ariation in antifungal prophylaxis strategies in lung transplantation. Transpl Infect Dis 2006;8(4):213–8.

40. Dauber JH, Paradis IL, Dummer JS. Infectious complications in pulmonary allograft recipients. Clin Chest Med 1990;11(2):291–308.

41. Duarte AG, Lick S. Perioperative care of lung transplant patients. Chest Surg Clin N Am 2002;12: 397–416.

42. Smyth TL, Scott JP, Borysiewicz LK, et al. Cytomegalovirus infection in heart-lung transplant recipients: risk factors, clinical associations, and response to treatment. J Infect Dis 1991;164(6): 1045–50.

43. Duncan SR, Grgurich WF, Iacono AT, et al. A comparison of ganciclovir and acyclovir to prevent cytomegalovirus after lung transplantation. Am J Respir Crit Care Med 1994;150(1):146–52.

44. Meyers BF, Lynch J, Trulock EP, et al. Lung transplantation: a decade of experience. Ann Surg 1999;230(3):362–70.

45. Calvo V, Borro JM, Morales P, et al. Antifungal prophylaxis during the early postoperative period of lung transplantation. Valencia Lung Transplant Group. Chest 1999;115(5):1301–4.

46. Morino E, Gallagher JC. Prophylactic antifungal agents used after lung transplantation. Ann Pharmacother 2010;44:546–56.

47. Reichenspurner H, Gamberg P, Nitschke M, et al. Significant reduction in the number of fungal infections after lung-, heart-lung, and heart transplantation using aerosolized amphotericin B prophylaxis. Transplant Proc 1997;29:627–8.

48. Minari A, Husni R, Avery RK, et al. The incidence of invasive aspergillosis among solid organ transplant recipients and implications for prophylaxis in lung transplants. Transpl Infect Dis 2002;4:195–200.

49. Husain S, Paterson DL, Studer S, et al. Voriconazole prophylaxis in lung transplant recipients. Am J Transplant 2006;6:3008–16.

50. Ramsey BW, Dorkin HL, Eisenberg JD, et al. Efficacy of aerosolized tobramycin in patients with cystic fibrosis. N Engl J Med 1993;328(24):1740–6.

51. Valerius NH, Koch C, Hoiby N. Prevention of chronic *Pseudomonas aeruginosa* colonisation in cystic fibrosis by early treatment. Lancet 1991;338(8769): 725–6.

52. Bauldoff GS, Nunley DR, Manzetti JD, et al. Use of aerosolized colistin sodium in cystic fibrosis patients awaiting lung transplantation. Transplantation 1997; 64(5):748–52.

53. Davies CW, Gleeson FV, Davies RJ. BTS guidelines for management of pleural infection. Thorax 2003; 58:ii18–28.

54. Alfageme I, Munoz F, Pena N, et al. Empyema of the thorax in adults. Etiology, microbiologic findings, and management. Chest 1993;103:839–43.

55. Sherman MM, Subramanian V, Berger RL. Management of thoracic empyema. Am J Surg 1977;133: 474–9.

56. Hughes CE, Van Scoy RE. Antibiotic therapy of pleural empyema. Semin Respir Infect 1991;6: 94–102.

57. Taryle DA, Good JT, Morgan EJ, et al. Antibiotic concentrations in human parapneumonic effusions. Antimicrob Agents Chemother 1981;7:171–7.

58. Huchon G, Woodhead M. Guidelines for management of adult community-acquired lower respiratory tract infections. European Study on Community-acquired Pneumonia (ESOCAP) Committee. Eur Respir J 1998;11:986.

Physiologic Evaluation of Lung Resection Candidates

Elizabeth A. David, MD[a], M. Blair Marshall, MD[b],*

KEYWORDS

- Lung resection • Physiologic evaluation
- Cardiovascular risk • Spirometry

Cure for patients with lung cancer is best achieved with surgical resection, but many lung cancers occur in patients who have abnormal pulmonary function typically due to cigarette smoking.[1] Alterations in normal pulmonary function and respiratory mechanics may limit a patient's recovery or quality of life after curative lung surgery, thus negating the benefit of curative resection. Therefore, careful analysis of patients' comorbidities and pulmonary function is a critical step when considering these patients for surgery. Each patient deserves a complete and individualized workup when being considered for lung resection, but there are many facets that the workup should include. Evidence-based guidelines are published by many of the thoracic societies, and should be used as a model for individual patient evaluations.[2–5]

The relationship between cigarette smoking and lung cancer is well established and, unfortunately, smoking itself predisposes these patients to many comorbid conditions, especially cardiovascular disease, which increases perioperative risk.[6] In patients with a significant history of smoking, it is particularly important to evaluate for concomitant cardiovascular disease prior to lung resection.

When considering patients for surgery, a balance must be reached between immediate perioperative risk and risk of long-term disability after lung resection. For patients in whom perioperative risk or long-term disability may be too high, nonsurgical therapies may be considered. Three-year follow-up of medically inoperable patients with stage 1 tumors treated with stereotactic body radiotherapy (SBRT), demonstrated local control rates of greater than 90% on Kaplan-Meier analysis, but longer-term follow-up is needed to demonstrate a true survival advantage over surgery.[7] It must be acknowledged that a decision between surgery and nonsurgical therapy is itself complicated at times. When individual patient risk factors are added to the scenario the decision can be overwhelming, and obtaining informed consent from patients can be a challenge. Multidisciplinary evaluation by a thoracic oncology team consisting of a thoracic surgeon, medical oncologist, radiation oncologist, and pulmonologist is helpful in risk assessment and can also be helpful in counseling patients for both surgical and nonsurgical therapy.[3] The thoracic surgeon, in deciding a patient is an acceptable operative risk, should bear the ultimate responsibility for the decision to perform surgery. Although not associated with a survival benefit, patients who undergo evaluation by a multidisciplinary team have better rates of treatment receipt for chemotherapy and radiation ($P<.001$ for both), but no difference in rates of surgical treatment.[8]

There are general factors that should be considered when optimizing patients for lung resection. A comprehensive history and physical examination should be performed, including but not limited to collecting data on age, comorbid disease including cardiovascular disease, and nutritional status. Most of the factors in an evaluation are patient related, but surgical-center experience and surgeon

The authors have nothing to disclose.
[a] University of Texas, MD Anderson Cancer Center, Houston, TX 77030, USA
[b] Division of Thoracic Surgery, Department of Surgery, Georgetown University Medical Center, 4 PHC, 3800 Reservoir Road, NW, Washington, DC 20007, USA
* Corresponding author.
E-mail address: Mbm5@gunet.georgetown.edu

specialty can play a role in surgical mortality and morbidity, and should be considered.[9] After this overall risk assessment is complete, evaluation of pulmonary function and cardiopulmonary exercise tolerance is necessary, and is described later.

AGE

In the past, age has been considered to increase perioperative risk and has been a reason to exclude surgery from therapeutic options for older patients. Patients older than 70 years are often poorly represented in clinical trials evaluating multimodality therapies, but recent surgical series have suggested that age alone is not a poor predictor of perioperative morbidity and mortality.[10,11] Okami and colleagues[11] described a series of 367 patients older than 80 years who underwent surgical resection for stage 1 non–small cell lung cancer (NSCLC), and reported an operative mortality of 1.4% and demonstrated that advanced pathologic state and comorbidities were independent predictors of decreased survival ($P<.0001$ and $P = .032$). Similarly, Birim and colleagues[12] found that in patients older than 70 years, comorbid disease rather than age was the most important influence on mortality. Patients should not be excluded from consideration for surgery on the basis of age alone (Level C evidence).

NUTRITION

As with any surgical procedure, the nutritional status of the patient is crucial for wound healing, avoidance of wound infection, and successful weaning from mechanical ventilator support.[4] Low preoperative prealbumin levels have been shown to correlate with increased postoperative complications.[13] Optimizing nutritional status before surgery is important in minimizing postoperative morbidity, but it is not mandatory to check prealbumin levels in patients for whom there is no clinical concern about nutritional status (Level C evidence).

CARDIOVASCULAR RISK

Cardiovascular disease is common among patients who smoke and who have lung cancer, therefore a careful cardiovascular risk assessment is a crucial part of an evaluation for lung resection. Because the mortality risks with cardiovascular disease are so high, it is essential that the American College of Cardiology (ACC) and American Heart Association (AHA) guidelines be followed for the evaluation of patients having noncardiac surgery.[14] When determining the appropriate cardiac evaluation, it is necessary to consider the following before initiating any invasive evaluation[15]:

- Clinical characteristics of the patient and comorbid disease
- The cardiac risk of the planned procedure
- The patient's functional status.

A change to the 2007 guidelines from the ACC/AHA includes an emphasis on the active cardiac conditions that must be addressed prior to surgery to prevent their manifestations from resulting in a significant delay in surgery.

The ACC and AHA have conveniently incorporated their screening workup into 5 questions for practitioners to guide evaluation for noncardiac surgery.

1. Is the surgery needed an emergency? If so, proceed with surgery, use heart rate control as clinical situation will allow, manage cardiac issues that arise expectantly. Do not delay life-saving surgery for perioperative cardiac workup.[14,15]
2. Is there an active cardiac condition, that is, heart failure, arrhythmias, valvular heart disease? If so, these should be assessed with electrocardiography (ECG), chest radiograph, and echocardiogram, and patients should be medically optimized as appropriate.[14,15]
3. What is the cardiac risk of the planned operation? Most operations except for vascular surgery, abdominal or thoracic surgery, head and neck surgery, orthopedic surgery, or prostate surgery are classified as low risk and carry a less than 1% risk of cardiac death or nonfatal myocardial infarction. Pulmonary resections are classified as intermediate risk procedures and carry a 1% to 5% risk of perioperative cardiac morbidity or mortality. Therefore, according to the ACC/AHA guidelines all patients having thoracic surgery must have an assessment of their functional status.[15]
4. What is the functional status of the patient? For the ACC/AHA guidelines, functional status is assessed with metabolic equivalent levels (MET). Strenuous activities typically require 10 METs and activities of daily living require 1 to 2 METs. Patients will need to be able to withstand 4 to 5 METs to tolerate the stress of noncardiac surgery under general anesthesia. If they are unable to tolerate this amount of exertion, consideration of specific clinical risk factors is needed before surgery.[14,15]
5. What are the patient's clinical risk factors? Risk factors including prior ischemic heart conditions and history of congestive heart failure, stroke, diabetes, or renal insufficiency, when present, necessitate further workup and

consultation with a cardiologist prior to decision making concerning operative risk. These patients will need appropriately monitored heart rate control in the perioperative period. Stress testing is not recommended for patients undergoing thoracic surgery who have 1 to 2 risk factors if they are receiving heart rate control. If stress testing is performed and demonstrates abnormal results, patients should be referred for percutaneous coronary intervention (PCI) or coronary artery bypass grafting (CABG). These interventions will delay the noncardiac surgery by 1 month for PCI and 6 to 8 weeks for CABG.[14,15]

For thoracic surgery, cardiac risk is acknowledged to be 1% to 5%, but postoperative surveillance of ischemic events is not currently recommended. When patients are clinically symptomatic, ECG and troponin measurements are recommended for detection of myocardial ischemia. For patients under consideration for lung cancer resection, these are intermediate-risk operations that will rarely be emergency procedures, therefore functional and cardiac risk factor assessment is warranted (Level B evidence).

SURGEON SPECIALTY

Schipper and colleagues[9] used data from the National Inpatient Sample (NIS) from 1996 to 2005 to show that general thoracic surgeons had significantly decreased the odds of death and lengths of stay greater than 14 days for lobectomy when compared with general surgeons. General thoracic surgeons were defined as those who perform more than 75% general thoracic operations and fewer than 10% cardiac operations. When adjusted for surgeon volume, the differences between specialties for differences in odds of death disappeared, but differences in length of stay persisted. Overall the investigators concluded that differences in morbidity are significantly affected by surgeon volume and specialty. Goodney and colleagues[16] also demonstrated decreased mortality for lung resections performed by thoracic surgeons as compared with general surgeons, using the national Medicare database from 1998 to 1999. These data suggest that experience of both the surgeon performing the procedure and the hospital should be considered in the evaluation of potential lung resection candidates (Level C evidence). Although surgeon specialty may not be formally considered part of the physiologic evaluation of the patient, given the decreased morbidity associated with pulmonary resection performed by a general thoracic surgeon, one should

consider this factor in the calculated risk for the patient, especially in marginal patients.

PULMONARY FUNCTION TESTING

After the completion of an overall risk assessment, specific measures of pulmonary function, including forced expiratory volume in 1 second (FEV_1) and diffusion capacity of carbon dioxide (DLCO), are essential. Depending on these results, further risk assessment may be performed with cardiopulmonary exercise testing and arterial blood gas measurements to completely evaluate a patient for pulmonary resection. When assessing pulmonary function, it is important to determine whether the patient will tolerate the operation and whether they will face a serious respiratory handicap after lung resection. Postoperative pulmonary function can be calculated in several different ways; including an estimation of the portion of remaining bronchopulmonary segments using FEV_1, calculation of the remaining lung function using estimation from a radionucleotide perfusion scan, or quantitative computed tomography (CT) scanning to estimate the remaining lung volumes after resection.[17]

Although these calculations are straightforward for the majority of patients, complex situations arise in relation to previous procedures or central disease whereby there may be alterations in ventilation of perfusion from obstruction by tumor. In these settings, a quantitative ventilation-perfusion (VQ) scan may provide additional information. Moreover, the multidisciplinary approach allows for the discussion of not only the impact of a potential planned surgical resection but also other modalities. At times, in patients with emphysema and poor pulmonary reserve, a limited anatomic resection may be associated with less anticipated risk than the standard radiation option, as this treatment modality is not without impact on pulmonary function.

SPIROMETRY

Measurement of FEV_1 is important for prediction of a patient's risk for postoperative complications and death. Both absolute values and predicted values are used for risk assessment, and it should be acknowledged that the degree of decrease in FEV_1 is inversely proportional to the degree of tumor-related obstruction. Historically, absolute values of FEV_1 greater than 1.5 L for lobectomy and greater than 2 L for pneumonectomy have been used as cutoff values, but it is acknowledged that predicted postoperative values as percentages of normal are more useful because they account for age, sex, and height.[17]

Predicted postoperative FEV_1 (PPO FEV_1) has been shown to be an independent predictor of perioperative mortality and morbidity.[18] In their study, Kearney used a PPO FEV_1 of less than 1 L as a marker for increased complications. In addition, they showed that for each decrease in PPO FEV_1 of 0.2 L, there was a 1.46 increased risk of complications (95% confidence interval 1.2–1.8). In other studies that have used PPO FEV_1 expressed as a percentage, PPO FEV_1 less than 40% was associated with increased rates of complications and death.[19–21]

Whereas many of the studies evaluating pulmonary function after lung resection have looked at patients who have undergone thoracotomy, fewer studies have looked at the differences between pulmonary function after thoracotomy and video-assisted thoracic surgery (VATS). In a series of 340 patients undergoing lobectomy via either thoracotomy or VATS, FEV_1 and DLCO were found to be significant predictors of morbidity for patients undergoing thoracotomy, but not in those undergoing VATS.[22] More studies are needed to determine the reasons for the varied effect on pulmonary function between the two operative techniques, but preservation of chest wall mechanics and decreased pain with a VATS approach may offer some explanation.

In addition to FEV_1, DLCO is a useful marker for operative risk. DLCO has been shown to have a higher correlation with postoperative death than PPO FEV_1. When the DLCO is less than 80% postoperative pulmonary complications are increased, and when the DLCO is less than 60%, there is increased postoperative mortality.[23] DLCO is not only important in assessing perioperative risk, but is also predictive of long-term survival after curative resection for lung cancer. In a study of 450 patients, DLCO less than 40% predicted decreased survival from causes other than lung cancer independently of FEV_1.[24] In patients who undergo induction chemotherapy, it is important to consider that DLCO is usually decreased by chemotherapeutic regimens and may worsen operative morbidity. In 66 patients who received induction chemotherapy, DLCO decreased by 21% and the predicted postoperative DLCO% (PPO DLCO%) was an independent risk factor for pulmonary complications.[25] In patients with congestive heart failure, the DLCO can be independently affected, and this must be considered as well.

TUMOR-RELATED ANATOMIC AND OTHER CONSIDERATIONS

In attempting to identify those patients at greatest risk and those who would not benefit from surgery, many data have been generated on the values of pulmonary performance and how they relate to the relative risk of a procedure. These parameters are applicable to the majority of patients; however, there are times when these values do not give the entire picture. Given the spectrum of the pathology that we treat along with our intimate understanding of the anatomy, thoracic surgeons are best suited to anticipate these complexities.

One cannot look at pulmonary performance and predictive postoperative values in isolation of the anatomic details associated with the pathologic process. Tumors that obstruct the airway may create a VQ mismatch, and this should be taken into consideration when evaluating patients for pulmonary resection. If a portion of a segment or lobe is partially or completely atelectatic, surgical resection may not have the anticipated negative impact on postoperative function. At times, one may even improve pulmonary function with resection by decreasing the VQ mismatch, given that the atelectatic parenchyma may be receiving no ventilation but full perfusion.

Encasement of the vessels by tumor may lead to decreased perfusion and another VQ mismatch. In this setting, a planned resection may not have as great an impact on pulmonary performance as it would if one went by the standard criteria. This factor comes into play when dealing with any obstruction, but may be most significant in the event of an anticipated pneumonectomy. In calculating the risk associated with a pneumonectomy, for instance, a planned right-sided pneumonectomy in a patient with 60% perfusion to the right lung may be more prone to postoperative complications than a patient with 15% perfusion to the right lung. In this setting in patients without any previous surgery, one may request a quantitative VQ study to more adequately calculate the impact of a planned resection on the postoperative predicted performance.

Alterations in the standard calculations may also be considered in the management of patients with severe emphysema. Given what has been learned from lung volume reduction surgery, some patients with poor lung function may actually derive a benefit from resection or, at least, the negative impact on performance may not be as traditionally calculated. Patients with upper lobe predominant emphysema and a corresponding lesion within the same lobe may tolerate surgery when it acts, in part, as a lung volume reduction procedure in addition to a cancer resection.

All patients under consideration for pulmonary resection should have pulmonary function assessed with spirometry. Patients who have PPO FEV_1 less than 40% and DLCO less than 40%

are at increased risk for perioperative morbidity and mortality, but these values should not be used as strict exclusion criteria from surgical therapy (Level C evidence).

CARDIOPULMONARY EXERCISE TESTING

Maximal oxygen consumption (Vo_{2max}) is measured during formal cardiopulmonary exercise testing (CPET), which records the exercise ECG, heart rate in response to exercise, minute ventilation, and oxygen uptake per minute.[3] CPET is a sophisticated physiologic test and is not available in all centers, but the stair-climbing test and shuttle-walk tests can be considered as adjuncts when formal CPET is not available. When Vo_{2max} is less than 15 mL/kg/min, patients are considered at high risk for surgery.[26] There is controversy over whether absolute Vo_{2max} is a better predictor of morbidity, but some investigators argue that Vo_{2max} expressed as a percentage of predicted normal values is a better predictor of poor surgical outcome.[26] Most centers agree that Vo_{2max} of 15 to 20 mL/kg/min or 50% to 60% of predicted is a safe cutoff for low postoperative mortality and morbidity.[26,27] Walsh and colleagues[27] reported a study of 66 patients undergoing pulmonary resection for NSCLC. In patients with a Vo_{2max} greater than 15 mL/kg/min there were no deaths but 40% of patients had complications; however, in patients with a Vo_{2max} less than 15 mL/kg/min there was a 20% mortality rate.

CPET allows for formal evaluation of the cardiopulmonary reserve that may be needed to survive the stress of surgery and its potential complications, therefore it is particularly useful in high-risk patients.[28] Critics of CPET argue that it can be limited in its ability to measure Vo_{2max} in patients who are unable to reach peak exertion because of other limiting comorbidities, but Kasikcioglu and colleagues[28] suggest that calculation of an oxygen uptake efficiency slope may allow for better prediction of surgical outcomes in patients with limited exercise capacity. CPET is usually recommended as an additional step when FEV_1 or DLCO is less than 40% of predicted postoperative lung function. Patients with Vo_{2max} of 10 to 15 mL/kg/min should be considered at high risk of perioperative morbidity and mortality after lung resection (Level C evidence).

STAIR CLIMBING

Stair climbing has been established as a reliable screening test of pulmonary function and a predictor of cardiopulmonary morbidity after lung resection.[29–31] Although there is wide variation in

administration of the test, generally patients are asked to walk up as many flights of stairs as possible, at their own pace, and to stop only for reasons of exhaustion, limiting dyspnea, leg fatigue, or chest pain, while being supervised by a health care professional. During the test heart rate, pulse oximetry, time, and height climbed are measured, and ergometric variables are calculated.[31] In general, the ability to climb 3 flights of stairs correlates with an FEV_1 of greater than 1.7 L and ability to tolerate a lobectomy; and 5 flights of stairs correlates with an FEV_1 of greater than 2 L, Vo_{2max} of greater than 20 mL/kg/min, and ability to tolerate pneumonectomy.[29,32]

Brunelli and colleagues[31] have demonstrated that patients who experience complications after lung resection are not able to climb as high as patients who do not experience complications ($P = .0004$). Patients who are unable to perform stair climbing because of comorbid conditions are at increased risk of death in the perioperative period after lung resection.[30] These data suggest that the stair-climbing test can be used as a surrogate for pulmonary function testing, as a predictor of cardiopulmonary morbidity after lung resection, and as a screening tool for patients under consideration for lung resection. Patients who are unable to complete 3 flights of stairs will be at increased risk of perioperative death and cardiopulmonary complications, and should be considered for nonsurgical therapy (Level C evidence).

SIX-MINUTE WALK TEST/SHUTTLE-WALK TEST

Two additional tests available as adjuncts for formal CPET are the 6-minute walk test and the shuttle-walk test.[3] The 6-minute walk test is rarely used because its predictive value for Vo_{2max} is limited and its interpretation is not standardized.[33] During the 6-minute walk test patients are asked to walk as far as they can, and rest periods are allowed. The 6-minute walk test is not currently recommended as a tool in the evaluation of potential lung resection candidates[33] (Level C evidence).

The shuttle-walk test requires that patients walk back and forth between two markers 10 m apart. The walking speed is set by an audio signal and is increased each minute of the test. The test is over when the patient is too short of breath to maintain the required speed. Unlike the 6-minute walk test, there is validation of the predictive value of the shuttle-walk test. Benzo and Sciurba showed that 50 patients with chronic obstructive pulmonary disease walking 25 shuttles correlated with a Vo_{2max} of greater than 15 mL/kg/min.[34] The shuttle-walk test can be used as an adjunct for formal CPET, but patients with borderline performance warrant further workup (Level C evidence).

ARTERIAL BLOOD GAS MEASUREMENTS

Arterial blood gas (ABG) analysis in the preoperative setting can be helpful in predicting postoperative morbidity. Arterial saturation (Sa_{O_2}) less than 90% is associated with increased postoperative complications.[35,36] In addition, hypercapnea ($PaCo_2$ >45 mm Hg) is associated with poor ventilatory function, but has not been shown to be an independent risk factor for postoperative death or higher complication rates.[37–39] Stein and colleagues[37] did demonstrate an increased risk of postoperative respiratory problems in patients with a $PaCo_2$ greater than 45 mm Hg. At present, in patients with Sa_{O_2} less than 90% or $PaCo_2$ greater than 45 mm Hg on preoperative ABG, additional evaluation should be completed prior to lung resection (Level C evidence).

ADDITIONAL CONSIDERATIONS
Risk of Long-Term Disability

Much of the evaluation of a candidate for pulmonary resection is spent on the assessment of perioperative risk, but it is also important to consider the long-term implications of lung resection on pulmonary function and exercise tolerance. Decreases in FEV_1 are seen following lung resection, but there is some recovery by the sixth postoperative month.[40] Studies have shown that actual FEV_1 is lower than PPO FEV_1, and actually worsens for the first 3 months after surgery with improvement by month 6.[40] Patients should be counseled about this expected fluctuation in pulmonary physiology, as this may be clinically symptomatic in patients with little reserve. In addition, in patients who will potentially receive induction chemotherapy, the lag time for improvement in FEV_1 may be up to 1 year.[41]

Patients may ask how symptomatic they will be after pulmonary resection, and this may be difficult to quantify. Leg discomfort rather than dyspnea is often an exercise-limiting symptom in these patients.[42] In addition, exercise capacity, as measured by stair climbing and 6-minute walk tests, unlike FEV_1, was not diminished after pulmonary resection in 40 patients.[43] When assessing a patient's risk of long-term disability, it is crucial to evaluate comorbid disease, predicted postoperative spirometry, cardiopulmonary exercise testing, and induction therapy to establish realistic patient expectations for the postoperative setting (Level C evidence).

Smoking Cessation

Accounting for regional differences, smoking remains common in patients with lung cancer, and the timing of smoking cessation is a frequent concern in the preoperative evaluation.[44] There is controversy over the best time interval to stop smoking prior to lung resection. Some studies suggest that at least 1 month smoke-free is needed before resection to minimize pulmonary complications, and other data suggest that there is no increased risk of pulmonary complications even with active smoking.[45,46] The Society of Thoracic Surgeons database was queried to determine the optimal time for smoking cessation prior to lung resection.[47] Among 7990 patients, smoking was found to increase the risk of hospital death and pulmonary complications, but there was no optimal time interval identified for smoking cessation before surgery.[47] However, because of the acknowledged risks of smoking concerning death and pulmonary complications, all patients should be counseled to stop smoking prior to lung resection regardless of the timing (Level B evidence).

Pulmonary Rehabilitation

Pulmonary rehabilitation in the preoperative setting has been controversial, but data extracted from the National Emphysema Treatment Trial (NETT) demonstrated a benefit for preoperative pulmonary rehabilitation.[48] All patients in the NETT received preoperative pulmonary rehabilitation and experienced less dyspnea, improved quality of life, and increased exercise tolerance. Preoperative pulmonary rehabilitation was thought to contribute to patients' preparation for lung volume reduction surgery, but there was no control group who did not receive preoperative pulmonary rehabilitation.[48] In a recent series from the Mayo clinic, 10 patients were randomized to a short duration of a customized protocol including exercise, inspiratory muscle training, and practice of slow breathing before lung resection.[49] These patients had shorter length of hospital stay ($P = .058$), fewer prolonged chest tubes ($P = .03$), and fewer days needing a chest tube ($P = .04$).[49] Based on these data, it is suggested that a customized preoperative pulmonary rehabilitation program may be feasible and efficacious in reducing perioperative morbidity (Level B/C evidence).

SUMMARY

After careful history and physical examination, patients under consideration for resection for lung cancer should undergo thorough physiologic evaluation and generalized risk assessment. Once data are available on comorbid disease, cardiovascular risk, pulmonary function, and exercise tolerance, they should be analyzed by a multidisciplinary team who will provide counseling regarding the risks, benefits, and alternatives to surgical and nonsurgical treatments for lung cancer. Anatomic contributions of tumor-related obstruction, both airway and vasculature, should be taken into consideration when calculating the impact of surgical resection. No patient should be excluded from consideration for surgical therapy based on one data point—a comprehensive evaluation is necessary for each patient. All patients should be counseled regarding smoking cessation.

REFERENCES

1. Kim SR, Han HJ, Park SJ, et al. Comparison between surgery and radiofrequency ablation for stage I non-small cell lung cancer. Eur J Radiol 2011. [Epub ahead of print].

2. Beckles MA, Spiro SG, Colice GL, et al. American College of Chest Physicians. The physiologic evaluation of patients with lung cancer being considered for resectional surgery. Chest 2003;123(Suppl 1): 105S–14S.

3. Colice GL, Shafazand S, Griffin JP, et al. American College of Chest Physicians. Physiologic evaluation of the patient with lung cancer being considered for resectional surgery: ACCP evidenced-based clinical practice guidelines (2nd edition). Chest 2007; 132(Suppl 3):161S–77S.

4. British Thoracic Society, Society of Cardiothoracic Surgeons of Great Britain and Ireland Working Party. BTS guidelines: guidelines on the selection of patients with lung cancer for surgery. Thorax 2001; 56(2):89–108.

5. Brunelli A, Charloux A, Bolliger CT, et al. The European Respiratory Society and European Society of Thoracic Surgeons clinical guidelines for evaluating fitness for radical treatment (surgery and chemoradiotherapy) in patients with lung cancer. Eur J Cardiothorac Surg 2009;36(1):181–4.

6. Krebs P, Coups EJ, Feinstein MB, et al. Health behaviors of early-stage non-small cell lung cancer survivors. J Cancer Surviv 2011. [Epub ahead of print].

7. Baumann P, Nyman J, Hoyer M, et al. Outcome in a prospective phase II trial of medically inoperable stage I non-small-cell lung cancer patients treated with stereotactic body radiotherapy. J Clin Oncol 2009;27(20):3290–6.

8. Boxer MM, Vinod SK, Shafiq J, et al. Do multidisciplinary team meetings make a difference in the management of lung cancer? Cancer 2011. [Epub ahead of print].

9. Schipper PH, Diggs BS, Ungerleider RM, et al. The influence of surgeon specialty on outcomes in general thoracic surgery: a national sample 1996 to 2005. Ann Thorac Surg 2009;88(5):1566–72 [discussion: 1572–3].

10. Pallis AG, Scarci M. Are we treating enough elderly patients with early stage non-small cell lung cancer? Lung Cancer 2011. [Epub ahead of print].

11. Okami J, Higashiyama M, Asamura H, et al. Japanese Joint Committee of Lung Cancer Registry. Pulmonary resection in patients aged 80 years or over with clinical stage I non-small cell lung cancer: prognostic factors for overall survival and risk factors for postoperative complications. J Thorac Oncol 2009;4(10):1247–53.

12. Birim O, Zuydendorp M, Maat AP, et al. Lung resection for non-small-cell lung cancer in patients older than 70. Ann Thorac Surg 2003;76:1796–801.

13. Bianchi RC, de Souza JN, de Giaciani AC, et al. Prognostic factors for complications following pulmonary resection: pre-albumin analysis, time on mechanical ventilation, and other factors. J Bras Pneumol 2006;32(6):489–94.

14. Fleisher LA, Beckman JA, Brown KA, et al. ACC/AHA 2007 guidelines on perioperative cardiovascular evaluation and care for noncardiac surgery: executive summary: a report of the American College of Cardiology/American Heart Association Task Force on Practice Guidelines (Writing Committee to Revise the 2002 Guidelines on Perioperative Cardiovascular Evaluation for Noncardiac Surgery). Anesth Analg 2008;106(3):685–712.

15. Freeman WK, Gibbons RJ. Perioperative cardiovascular assessment of patients undergoing noncardiac surgery. Mayo Clin Proc 2009;84(1):79–90.

16. Goodney PP, Lucas FL, Stukel TA, et al. Surgeon specialty and operative mortality with lung resection. Ann Surg 2005;241(1):179–84.

17. Poonyagariyagorn H, Mazzone PJ. Lung cancer: preoperative pulmonary evaluation of the lung resection candidate. Semin Respir Crit Care Med 2008;29(3):271–84.

18. Kearney DJ, Lee TH, Reilly JJ, et al. Assessment of operative risk in patients undergoing lung resection. Importance of predicted pulmonary function. Chest 1994;105(3):753–9.

19. Brunelli A, Fianchini A. Predicted postoperative FEV1 and complications in lung resection candidates. Chest 1997;111(4):1145–6.

20. Putnam JB Jr, Lammermeier DE, Colon R, et al. Predicted pulmonary function and survival after pneumonectomy for primary lung carcinoma. Ann Thorac Surg 1990;49(6):909–14 [discussion: 915].

21. Nakahara K, Ohno K, Hashimoto J, et al. Prediction of postoperative respiratory failure in patients undergoing lung resection for lung cancer. Ann Thorac Surg 1988;46(5):549–52.

22. Berry MF, Villamizar-Ortiz NR, Tong BC, et al. Pulmonary function tests do not predict pulmonary complications after thoracoscopic lobectomy. Ann Thorac Surg 2010;89(4):1044–51 [discussion: 1051–2].

23. Ferguson MK, Little L, Rizzo L, et al. Diffusing capacity predicts morbidity and mortality after pulmonary resection. J Thorac Cardiovasc Surg 1988;96(6):894–900.

24. Liptay MJ, Basu S, Hoaglin MC, et al. Diffusion lung capacity for carbon monoxide (DLCO) is an independent prognostic factor for long-term survival after curative lung resection for cancer. J Surg Oncol 2009;100(8):703–7.

25. Takeda S, Funakoshi Y, Kadota Y, et al. Fall in diffusing capacity associated with induction therapy for lung cancer: a predictor of postoperative complication? Ann Thorac Surg 2006;82(1):232–6.

26. Win T, Jackson A, Sharples L, et al. Cardiopulmonary exercise tests and lung cancer surgical outcome. Chest 2005;127(4):1159–65.

27. Walsh GL, Morice RC, Putnam JB Jr, et al. Resection of lung cancer is justified in high-risk patients selected by exercise oxygen consumption. Ann Thorac Surg 1994;58(3):704–10 [discussion: 711].

28. Kasikcioglu E, Toker A, Tanju S, et al. Oxygen uptake kinetics during cardiopulmonary exercise testing and postoperative complications in patients with lung cancer. Lung Cancer 2009;66(1):85–8.

29. Bolton JW, Weiman DS, Haynes JL, et al. Stair climbing as an indicator of pulmonary function. Chest 1987;92(5):783–8.

30. Brunelli A, Al Refai M, Monteverde M, et al. Stair climbing test predicts cardiopulmonary complications after lung resection. Chest 2002;121(4):1106–10.

31. Brunelli A, Monteverde M, Al Refai M, et al. Stair climbing test as a predictor of cardiopulmonary complications after pulmonary lobectomy in the elderly. Ann Thorac Surg 2004;77(1):266–70.

32. Pollock M, Roa J, Benditt J, et al. Estimation of ventilatory reserve by stair climbing. A study in patients with chronic airflow obstruction. Chest 1993;104(5):1378–83.

33. Brunelli A, Pompili C, Salati M. Low-technology exercise test in the preoperative evaluation of lung resection candidates. Monaldi Arch Chest Dis 2010;73(2):72–8.

34. Benzo RP, Sciurba FC. Oxygen consumption, shuttle walking test and the evaluation of lung resection. Respiration 2010;80(1):19–23.

35. Chetta A, Tzani P, Marangio E, et al. Respiratory effects of surgery and pulmonary function testing in the preoperative evaluation. Acta Biomed 2006;77(2):69–74.

36. Turner SE, Eastwood PR, Cecins NM, et al. Physiologic responses to incremental and self-paced exercise in COPD: a comparison of three tests. Chest 2004;126(3):766–73.

37. Stein M, Koota GM, Simon M, et al. Pulmonary evaluation of surgical patients. JAMA 1962;181:765–70.

38. Morice RC, Peters EJ, Ryan MB, et al. Exercise testing in the evaluation of patients at high risk for complications from lung resection. Chest 1992;101(2):356–61.

39. Harpole DH, Liptay MJ, DeCamp MM Jr, et al. Prospective analysis of pneumonectomy: risk factors for major morbidity and cardiac dysrhythmias. Ann Thorac Surg 1996;61(3):977–82.

40. Nezu K, Kushibe K, Tojo T, et al. Recovery and limitation of exercise capacity after lung resection for lung cancer. Chest 1998;113(6):1511–6.

41. Funakoshi Y, Takeda S, Sawabata N, et al. Long-term pulmonary function after lobectomy for primary lung cancer. Asian Cardiovasc Thorac Ann 2005;13(4):311–5.

42. Bolliger CT, Jordan P, Solèr M, et al. Pulmonary function and exercise capacity after lung resection. Eur Respir J 1996;9(3):415–21.

43. Pancieri MV, Cataneo DC, Montovani JC, et al. Comparison between actual and predicted postoperative stair-climbing test, walk test and spirometric values in patients undergoing lung resection. Acta Cir Bras 2010;25(6):535–40.

44. Raupach T, Quintel M, Hinterthaner M. Preoperative smoking cessation in patients with lung cancer. Pneumologie 2010;64(11):694–700 [in German].

45. Nakagawa M, Tanaka H, Tsukuma H, et al. Relationship between the duration of the preoperative smoke-free period and the incidence of postoperative pulmonary complications after pulmonary surgery. Chest 2001;120(3):705–10.

46. Barrera R, Shi W, Amar D, et al. Smoking and timing of cessation: impact on pulmonary complications after thoracotomy. Chest 2005;127(6):1977–83.

47. Mason DP, Subramanian S, Nowicki ER, et al. Impact of smoking cessation before resection of lung cancer: a Society of Thoracic Surgeons General Thoracic Surgery Database study. Ann Thorac Surg 2009;88(2):362–70 [discussion 370–1].

48. Fishman A, Martinez F, Naunheim K, et al. National Emphysema Treatment Trial Research Group. A randomized trial comparing lung-volume-reduction surgery with medical therapy for severe emphysema. N Engl J Med 2003;348(21):2059–73.

49. Benzo R, Wigle D, Novotny P, et al. Preoperative pulmonary rehabilitation before lung cancer resection: results from two randomized studies. Lung Cancer 2011. [Epub ahead of print].

Management of Early Stage Non–Small Cell Lung Cancer in High-Risk Patients

Jessica S. Donington, MD[a],*, Justin D. Blasberg, MD[b]

KEYWORDS

- Non-small cell lung cancer • Sublobar resection
- Stereotactic body radiotherapy • Radiofrequency ablation

Between 20% and 25% of patients diagnosed with non–small cell lung cancer (NSCLC) have clinical stage I disease. Lobectomy with systematic mediastinal lymph node evaluation has been the accepted standard treatment of early-stage NSCLC since the 1940s. However, up to 20% of patients have limited pulmonary reserve.[1] Before 1995, treatment in this population was restricted to sublobar resection, conventionally fractionated radiation therapy (CFRT), or supportive care. Several nonsurgical treatment modalities have recently been introduced, including stereotactic body radiation therapy (SBRT) and percutaneous ablative therapy (radiofrequency ablation [RFA], cryotherapy [CRYO], and microwave [MWA] ablation). Although these treatments appear to decrease the risk of respiratory failure, disability, and death, there is limited evidence for efficacy compared with lobectomy. Furthermore, the morbidity and mortality associated with lobectomy has changed with time, particularly with the adoption of minimally invasive techniques. Untreated stage I NSCLC has a 1-year survival of 80%, which declines rapidly by 3 years after diagnosis.[2] Despite high competitive mortality from severe underlying lung disease, mortality related to untreated stage I NSCLC cannot be ignored except in the most debilitated patients.

In the past 15 years, there have been major improvements in radiographic technology, allowing for detection of smaller lesions and improved preprocedural staging. Balancing the risk of lobectomy against parenchymal-sparing resection or nonsurgical procedures is of great importance in frail patients. Evidence for assessment of interventional risk is covered in a separate article. The Evidence-Based Workforce of the Society of Thoracic Surgeons and the Thoracic Oncology Network of the American College of Chest Physicians recently undertook a systematic review of treatment of high-risk patients with stage I NSCLC.[3] This article provides a synopsis of that review, and the management suggestions are outlined in **Table 1**.

SUBLOBAR RESECTION

Sublobar resection has been a treatment option for stage I NSCLC for many decades. Early experience revealed comparable morbidity and reduced mortality,[4,5] with preservation of pulmonary function compared with lobectomy for early-stage disease.[6] When the Lung Cancer Study Group (LCSG) showed a threefold increase in regional recurrence (17.2% vs 6.4%) following sublobar resection compared with lobectomy, enthusiasm for this approach waned.[7] However, in the 2 decades since the LCSG trial, advancements in radiographic technology used to detect and diagnose NSCLC improved comprehension

a Department of Cardiothoracic Surgery, NYU School of Medicine, 530 1st Avenue, Suite 9V, New York, NY 10016, USA
b Department of Cardiothoracic Surgery, Massachusetts General Hospital, 55 Fruit Street, Blake 1570, Boston, MA 02114, USA
* Corresponding author.
E-mail address: jessica.donington@nyumc.org

Thorac Surg Clin 22 (2012) 55–65
doi:10.1016/j.thorsurg.2011.08.018
1547-4127/12/$ – see front matter © 2012 Elsevier Inc. All rights reserved.

<table>
<tr><td colspan="2">

Table 1
Summary of management suggestions from the STS/ACCP consensus statement on the treatment of high-risk stage I NSCLC[3]

</td></tr>
</table>

Sublobar resection	Segmentectomy or extended wedge resection with clear margins and hilar and mediastinal nodal sampling may represent a safe and effective alternative to lobectomy in high-risk patients with stage I NSCLC
	Segmentectomy or extended wedge resection can be effective and potentially beneficial in patients greater than 75 years of age with stage I NSCLC
	Anatomic segmentectomy may be beneficial compared with wedge resection in patients undergoing sublobar resection for stage I NSCLC
	Surgical margin >1 cm or equal to the tumor diameter is preferred when performing sublobar resection for stage I NSCLC
	Adjuvant intraoperative brachytherapy in conjunction with sublobar resection is associated with local and regional recurrence similar to that reported after lobectomy
Radiation therapy	CFRT with definitive intent and sufficient dose intensity is a treatment option for high-risk patients with stage I NSCLC
	In tumors <5 cm, where normal tissue dose constraints can be respected, SBRT is appropriate and preferred to CFRT for definitive treatment of high-risk stage I NSCLC
	A modified SBRT treatment schedule is recommended for tumors within 2 cm of the proximal bronchial tree
Percutaneous ablative therapy	RFA is a reasonable treatment option in high-risk patients with stage I NSCLC with peripheral lesions <3 cm. There is no consensus on treatment duration or number of treatments
	RFA in combination with conventionally fractionated radiation therapy may be considered for tumors >3 cm. There is no consensus on sequence of therapy
	RFA is not indicated for lesions adjacent to major bronchovascular structures, or esophagus

of tumor biology, and an increased prevalence of elderly and medically unfit patients with NSCLC has resurrected interest in sublobar resection. Numerous single-institution series have shown equivalent morbidity, mortality, regional recurrence, and survival for anatomic segmentectomy compared with lobectomy for small peripheral tumors (**Table 2**).[8–12] A prospective, randomized, multi-institutional study is currently being conducted by the Cancer and Leukemia Group B (140503) readdressing the comparison between sublobar resection and lobectomy for stage I NSCLC. This trial does not specifically target high-risk patients, but the implications for this group are significant.

Extent of Resection

Sublobar resections can be performed by anatomic segmentectomy or simple wedge resection. Segmentectomy follows anatomic planes and includes a wider resection of draining lymphatics, commonly referenced as a residual cancer cell basin.[13] Wedge resections are typically performed by stapling across parenchyma, not along anatomic planes, and are preferred because of their technical ease and speed of completion. In the LCSG, segmental resection had a decreased risk of involved lobe recurrence compared with wedge resection,[7] and more closely approximated recurrence and survival following lobectomy. Data suggest that wedge resection is an inferior oncologic approach compared with segmentectomy; Okada and colleagues[14] reported superior 5-year survival for segmentectomy compared with wedge resection. El-Sherif and colleagues[15] also noted higher involved lobe and regional recurrence with wedge compared with segmentectomy in 81 patients with stage I NSCLC. However, a strict definition for adequate margins remains unresolved; studies suggest that involved lobe and regional recurrence is decreased with margins greater than 1 cm or greater than the maximum tumor diameter.[15–17]

Tumor Size

Tumor size is important to the efficacy of sublobar resection. Several reports document equivalent disease-free survival when comparing lobectomy and segmentectomy for tumors less than or equal

Table 2
Comparisons of morbidity, mortality, local/regional recurrence, and survival between lobectomy and sublobar resection

Author	Year	Study Design	Lobectomy					Sublobar Resection				
			n	Morbidity (%)	Mortality (%)	Regional Recurrence (%)	5-Year Survival (%)	n	Morbidity (%)	Mortality (%)	Regional Recurrence (%)	5-Year Survival (%)
Ginsberg and Rubinstein[7]	1995	Prospective randomized	122	N/R	1.6	6.4	65	125	N/R	0.8	17	44
Landreneau et al[9]	1997	Prospective nonrandomized	117	31	3.3	9	68	102	21	0	19.6	58
Koike et al[8]	2003	Prospective nonrandomized	159	N/R	N/R	1.3	90.1	74	N/R	N/R	2.7	89.1
Martin-Ucar et al[10]	2005	Retrospective case matched	17	17.6	5.8	12	64	17	17.6	5.8	0	70
Okada et al[11]	2006	Prospective nonrandomized	305	6.6	N/R	4.9 (local, not further defined)	89.1	262	7.3	0.4	6.9 (local, not further defined)	89.6
Schuchert et al[12]	2007	Retrospective	246	32.4	3.3	4.9	80	182	33.7	1.1	7.7	83

Abbreviation: N/R, not recorded.

to 2 cm.[14,18,19] In a series of 1272 patients from Okada, no difference in disease-free survival following lobectomy or segmentectomy was noted for tumors less than or equal to 2 cm.[14] Reports examining sublobar resection for subcentimeter tumors also document no difference in involved lobe recurrence or survival between lobectomy and segmentectomy.[10,11] These findings mirror data from the recent lung cancer staging project by the International Association for the Study of Lung Cancer with respect to the importance of stratifying tumors around a 2 cm cutoff.[20] The ongoing Cancer and Leukemia Group B (CALGB) 140503 trial, evaluating sublobar resection to lobectomy, is limited to tumors less than or equal to 2 cm.

Impact of Age

Advanced age is associated with risk for morbidity and mortality following lung resection.[21] Several studies have explored the usefulness of sublobar resection for stage I NSCLC in the elderly. Data from the Surveillance, Epidemiology and End Results (SEER) Program showed no survival difference in patients more than 75 years old undergoing lobectomy or sublobar resection.[22] Kilic and colleagues[16] also noted reduced morbidity and mortality for patients more than 75 years old with stage I NSCLC who underwent segmentectomy compared with lobectomy, with no difference in regional recurrence or survival.

Adjuvant Brachytherapy

Brachytherapy can be used to decrease involved lobe recurrence following sublobar resection. Advantages of brachytherapy include increased convenience and assurance of delivery; poor compliance was an issue in a CALGB trial for external beam radiation after sublobar resection.[23,24] Single-institution series report decreased involved lobe recurrence, from 17.2% to 3.3%, with brachytherapy following sublobar resection.[19] Involved lobe and regional failures ranging from 2% to 6% with the addition of brachytherapy,[19,25–27] and compare favorably with the 6.4% involved lobe and regional recurrence following lobectomy in the LCSG.[7] The American College of Surgeons Oncology Group (ACOSOG) recently completed accrual on a prospective randomized trial (Z4032) comparing sublobar resection alone or with intraoperative brachytherapy for high-risk stage I patients with tumors less than 3 cm. No significant change from baseline pulmonary function tests (PFTs) was seen in either arm 3 months after resection.[28] Mortality was 2.7% at 90 days, and no difference in adverse events was noted between treatment groups.[29] Survival and recurrence data are maturing.

Summary

For select high-risk patients with stage I NSCLC, sublobar resection provides a parenchymal-sparing alternative to lobectomy. The use of segmentectomy may be particularly useful for peripheral tumors less than 2 cm located within anatomic segmental boundaries. Adjuvant intraoperative brachytherapy may reduce involved lobe recurrence following resection. The importance of adequate hilar and mediastinal staging cannot be overemphasized to avoid erroneous downstaging. Prospective, randomized studies (CALGB 140503 and ACOSOG Z4032) will better delineate the usefulness of sublobar resection in NSCLC.

RADIATION THERAPY
CFRT

Trials evaluating CFRT in patients with early-stage NSCLC with medical contraindications to resection indicate a modest prolongation of survival compared with observation alone and suggest the potential for cure in select patients.[30–32] A recent review of 18 studies using CFRT for NSCLC, including 1562 patients with medically inoperable stage I disease, showed an overall survival of 34%, and cancer-specific survival of 39% at 3 years.[33] Primary tumor relapse occurred in 40% and was the predominant cause of treatment failure. Modern CFRT techniques and dose intensification have improved outcomes, however 5-year involved lobe and regional control remains less than or equal to 70% and overall survival continues to be suboptimal.[34–36]

SBRT

SBRT refers to precise and accurate delivery of conformal and dose-intensive radiation to a small target. It requires computerized treatment planning, precise tumor tracking, and multiple transecting beams that allow for a steep decrease of radiation outside the treatment volume. SBRT has been available for intracranial tumors since 1990; techniques for intrathoracic tumors were first described by Blomgren and colleagues[37] in 1995. Multiple large phase II studies (**Table 3**)[38–52] show a dose-response relationship favoring more intensive regimens, and report higher rates of primary tumor control for smaller tumors. Regimes with biologic effective dose (BED) more than 100 Gy consistently report primary tumor control of more than 90% for T1 tumors and more than 85% in series including T2

Table 3
Prospective single-institution and multicenter/cooperative group studies evaluating SBRT for biopsy proven clinical stage I NSCLC

Author	N (% Medically Inoperable)	Nominal Dose	BED (Gy)	Primary Tumor Control	Overall Survival	Cancer-Specific Survival	Toxicity ≥Grade 3 (%)
Fukumoto et al[42]	22 (86)	48–60 Gy/8 fx	67–105	94% (2 y)	45% (2 y)	73% (2 y)	0
Onishi et al[48]	35 (66)	60 Gy/10 fx	96	94% (2 y)	58% (2 y)	83% (2 y)	0
McGarry et al[46]	47 (100)	24–72 Gy/3 fx	43–245	78% (2 y)	N/R	N/R	15
Yoon et al[52]	21 (76)	30 Gy/3 fx or 40–48 Gy/4 fx	60–106	81% (2 y)	51% (2 y)	86% (2 y)	0
Xia et al[51]	25 (100)	50 Gy/10 fx	75	96% (3 y)	91% (3 y)	N/R	4
Le et al[44]	22 (82)	15–30 Gy/1 fx	37.5–120	T1: 100% ≤20 Gy: 50% >20 Gy: 87%	46% (2 y)	62% (2 y)	13.5
Collins et al[40]	15 (100)	45–60 Gy/3 fx	112–180	100% (crude)	87% (2 y)	N/R (2 y)	6.5
Koto et al[43]	31 (65)	45 Gy/3 fx or 60 Gy/8 fx	112–105	T1 78% T2 40% (3 y)	72% (3 y)	83% (3 y)	6.5
Onimaru et al[47]	41 (85)	40–48 Gy/4 fx	80–105.6	73% (2 y)	64% (2 y)	73% (2 y)	5
Fakiris et al[41]	70 (100)	T1-60 Gy/3 fx T2-66 Gy/3 fx	180–211.2	88% (3 y)	43% (3 y)	82% (3 y)	15.7
Matsuo et al[45]	101 (63)	48 Gy/4 fx	105.6	87% (3 y)	59% (3 y)	N/R	5
Bauman et al[39] Nordic Study Group	57 (93)*	45 Gy/3 fx	112.5	92% (3 y)	60% (3 y)	88% (3 y)	30
Timmerman et al[50] RTOG 0236	55 (100)	60 Gy/3 fx	180	98% (3 y)	56% (3 y)	N/R	27

Abbreviations: BED, biologic equivalent dose; F/U, follow-up; fx, fraction; N/R, not recorded; RTOG, Radiation Therapy Oncology Group.
* 67% biopsy proven.

tumors. Overall survival is typically more than 50% in predominately medically unfit populations, which is superior to results from CFRT. A recent meta-analysis confirmed significant improvement in survival with SBRT compared with CFRT.[53]

The Radiation Therapy Oncology Group (RTOG) recently reported a prospective multi-institutional trial (RTOG 0236) limited to high-risk patients with stage I NSCLC treated with SBRT.[50] All patients had biopsy confirmation of the diagnosis, staging with computed tomography (CT)/positron emission tomography (PET), and were deemed medically inoperable by a thoracic surgeon or pulmonologist. Primary tumor control of 98%, regional control of 87%, and overall survival of 56% at 3 years were achieved. A subsequent trial, RTOG 0618, used the same treatment regimen but was limited to operative candidates. This trial completed accrual with outcome results maturing.

Toxicity

Treatment-related toxicity increases with dose, although high-grade toxicity is uncommon and treatment-related deaths rare. Reported toxicities include pneumonitis, fibrosis, dyspnea, rib fracture, chest wall pain, brachial plexopathy, dermatitis, skin ulceration, esophagitis, fistulas, and fatigue. Other factors contributing to toxicity include organ volume, prior thoracic radiotherapy, and radiosensitizing chemotherapy. Most trials report no significant change in PFTs following SBRT,[39,42,44] although 1 reported a mild decline in DLCO.[54] A study from Timmerman and colleagues[55] reported excessive toxicity in the treatment of tumors within 2 cm of the proximal bronchial tree, compared with peripheral tumors (46% vs 17% $\geq$ grade 3 toxicity at 2 years). Although central toxicity rates are not consistently observed with less intense SBRT regimens, caution is warranted when treating central lesions. RTOG 0913 is currently evaluating toxicity of less intensive regimes for central tumors.

Summary

For high-risk patients with stage I NSCLC, definitive radiation therapy is a treatment option with curative potential. A large volume of nonrandomized evidence recommends SBRT rather than CFRT because of superior survival and local tumor control. Two multicenter randomized trials underway in Scandinavia and Australia should provide definitive comparisons of these techniques. RTOG and ACOSOG (Z0499/1021) are sponsoring a randomized comparison of SBRT and sublobar resection for high-risk patients with stage I NSCLC. Simultaneously, 2 international phase III studies of

SBRT compared with lobectomy for operable patients, the Lung Cancer Stereotactic Radiotherapy vs Surgery (STARS) and Radiosurgery Or Surgery for Early Lung cancer (ROSEL) are ongoing. These trials should help define the ongoing use of this technology in stage I NSCLC.

PERCUTANEOUS ABLATIVE THERAPIES

Percutaneous ablation is an evolving technology for NSCLC treatment. There are 3 recognized modalities: RFA, MWA, and CRYO, with RFA being the most widely studied to date. All are catheter based and typically performed under CT guidance. There are no randomized control trials comparing direct lung ablation with SBRT or surgery, but evidence is accumulating that lung RFA is safe and feasible for the treatment of medically unresectable stage I NSCLC.[56–64] Three technologies are approved by the US Food and Drug Administration (FDA) for soft tissue RFA are available: RITA Medical Systems (Moutainview, CA, USA), Covidien (Valley Lab Division, Boulder, CO, USA), and Boston Scientific (Natick, MA, USA). Multiple expandable thermal electrodes are used with Boston Scientific and RITA, whereas an internally cooled electrode is used in the Covidien system. The efficacies of different systems have not been formally compared and there is no consensus regarding superiority. Treatment success depends on temperature; coagulation necrosis is achieved at temperatures of more than 60°C. Limitations of RFA include large tumor size and proximity to bronchovascular structures, esophagus, or trache. Tumors larger than 3 cm or within 1 cm of hilar structures are at risk for incomplete ablation and bronchovascular damage following RFA.[65]

Local and Regional Control

The level of evidence is low, with no randomized or case-control trials comparing RFA with conventional therapy for inoperable patients. Many studies include both primary and metastatic lung lesions, making it difficult to quantify the effect for NSCLC. Nine studies report specifically on outcomes for stage I NSCLC,[56,59–63,66–68] with a primary tumor relapse rate between 8% and 43% (**Table 4**).[56,57,59–63,68] Tumors larger than 3 cm were associated with primary tumor recurrence rates of more than 50%[58,60,68]; primary tumor relapse was improved to 8% to 12% with the addition of CFRT.[58,67]

Toxicity

Morbidity following RFA ranges from 15% to 55%[59–61,66–68]; pneumothorax (16%–54%) and

Table 4
Primary tumor control, survival, and toxicity following RFA for stage I NSCLC

Author	n	System	Median Tumor Size in cm (max)	Primary Tumor Control	Survival Overall	Survival Cancer Specific	Toxicity Pneumothorax (%)	Toxicity Chest Tube (%)	Toxicity Pleural Effusion (%)
Lee et al[61]	10	Covidien	4.1 (6)	60% (1 y)	80% (1 y)	100% (1 y)	35	7	7
Belfiore et al[66]	33	Covidien/RITA	3.5 (6)	N/R	N/R	N/R	9	0	9
Pennathur et al[63]	19	RITA	2.6 (3.8)	58% (2 y)	68% (2 y)	N/R	63	63	N/R
Dupuy et al[67]	24	Covidien +66 Gy CFRT	3.5 (7.5)	N/R	N/R	N/R	29	12	N/R
Hiraki et al[68]	20	Covidien/Boston Scientific	2.4 (6)	63% (3 y)	74% (3 y)	83% (3 y)	57	5	17
Hsie et al[59]	12	Boston Scientific	N/R	92% (3 y)	50% (3 y)	N/R	25	25	N/R
Beland et al[56]	69	Covidien	2.5 (5)	62% (2 y)	N/R	30% (3 y)	N/R	N/R	N/R
Lanuti et al[60]	31	Covidien	2 (4.4)	68.% (3 y)	47% (3 y)	39% (3 y)	13	8	21
Lencioni[62]	13	RITA	1.5 (3.4)	87.% (2 y)	75% (2 y)	92% (2 y)	N/R	N/R	N/R
Fernando et al[57]	9	Boston Scientific	2.5 (4.5)	66% (2 y)	N/R	N/R	N/R	N/R	N/R

Abbreviations: F/U, follow-up; max, maximum reported tumor size; N/R, not reported.

pleural effusion (∼19%) are most common (see **Table 4**). Other complications include bronchopleural fistula, massive hemoptysis, hemothorax, neuropathy, and pneumonia.[60,69,70] Procedure-related mortality is less than 1%; however, RFA in patients with previous pneumonectomy has been associated with death in 2 series.[64,71] Several publications report no significant loss in lung function.[60,72,73]

Cancer-specific Survival

Five-year survival has not been sufficiently evaluated. Two-year cancer-specific survival ranges from 57% to 93%.[60,62,68] Overall 1-year, 2-year, and 3-year survival has been reported as 63% to 85%, 55% to 65%, and 15% to 46% (see **Table 4**).[70] An ongoing phase I/II trial from ACOSOG (Z4033) addresses the uniformity of RFA treatment in high-risk stage I NSCLC. Primary objectives are 2-year survival and freedom from local/regional recurrence. The trial also evaluates the role for early PET in predicting primary tumor control, and explores short-term and long-term effects of RFA on PFTs. This study has completed accrual, and survival data are maturing. PET obtained within 96 hours of treatment was not found to be helpful in predicting response to therapy.[74]

Alternative Ablative Therapies

The clinical efficacy of CRYO and MWA for NSCLC is poorly defined to date, with only a few observational series published.[75,76] CRYO is performed using an argon-helium–based system (Endocare, Irvine, CA, USA); treatment involves a freeze-thaw-refreeze cycle ranging from 15 to 60 minutes, based on tumor size. As with RFA, the peripheral zone has limited cytotoxicity and therefore 3-mm to 5-mm margins are recommended. One advantage of CRYO is safety for central lesions because of the preservation of collagenous structures.[77] MWA is a thermal-based system, coagulating via electromagnetic waves, with a theoretic advantage of generating higher temperatures and steeper tissue drop-off compared with RFA. However, both technologies far are less established than RFA.

SUMMARY

NSCLC has a strong tendency for early metastatic spread and therefore presents a management challenge for localized therapy even in early-stage disease. Lobectomy with systematic mediastinal lymph node evaluation is associated with excellent rates of local and regional control, but is not an option for all patients. Initial evidence

with SBRT, RFA, and sublobar resection showed an increased risk for local and regional recurrence, and inferior survival compared with lobectomy. However, use of these alternative techniques has been limited to frail populations and single-institution series, making direct comparisons with lobectomy difficult. Increased sensitivity of radiographic technology has allowed for detection of smaller/less aggressive cancers and improved the accuracy of pretreatment staging. Emerging evidence now suggests that, in well-staged and properly selected patients, sublobar resection, SBRT, and RFA may provide an equivalent curative option with decreased risk of periprocedural complications and death.

The biggest obstacle in direct comparisons of efficacy and safety of these modalities is the lack of commonality in the definitions for pretreatment medical evaluation, follow-up, response, and relapse between trials. Most current evidence is retrospective or from single-institution prospective evaluations, with only a handful of multi-institutional trials. Although there is some consistency in evaluation and outcome reporting within a given treatment modality, there is almost none across modalities. A common language and criteria for evaluation needs to be a priority. Simply stating that a patient is medically unfit to undergo lobectomy is inadequate; disability needs to be qualified and quantified to allow for appropriate comparisons between technologies. Similarly, outcomes are not defined by response or survival alone, but should include toxicity, cause of death, relapse location, and quality of life. Well-recognized and validated reporting criteria exist for these parameters, but collection and reporting has not been consistent.

A multidisciplinary approach is essential for the management of these patients, and a similar approach is needed on an organizational level to further define appropriate use of each modality. In the next decade, ongoing phase II and III trials may determine the superiority of one modality for high-risk populations. The inclusion of uniform preprocedural staging, medical assessment, and reporting of response, toxicity, recurrence, and quality of life is essential when comparing outcomes across treatment modalities.

REFERENCES

1. Mentzer SJ, Swanson SJ. Treatment of patients with lung cancer and severe emphysema. Chest 1999; 116:477S–9S.
2. Vrdoljak E, Mise K, Sapunar D, et al. Survival analysis of untreated patients with non-small-cell lung cancer. Chest 1994;106:1797–800.

3. Donington J, Ferguson M, Mazzone P, et al. STS/ACCP Consensus statement on evaluation and management for high risk patients with stage I non-small cell lung cancer. In; 2011.

4. Jensik RJ, Faber LP, Milloy FJ, et al. Segmental resection for lung cancer. A fifteen-year experience. J Thorac Cardiovasc Surg 1973;66:563–72.

5. Wada H, Nakamura T, Nakamoto K, et al. Thirty-day operative mortality for thoracotomy in lung cancer. J Thorac Cardiovasc Surg 1998;115:70–3.

6. Keenan RJ, Landreneau RJ, Maley RH Jr, et al. Segmental resection spares pulmonary function in patients with stage I lung cancer. Ann Thorac Surg 2004;78:228–33 [discussion: 233].

7. Ginsberg RJ, Rubinstein LV. Randomized trial of lobectomy versus limited resection for T1 N0 non-small cell lung cancer. Lung Cancer Study Group. Ann Thorac Surg 1995;60:615–22 [discussion: 22–3].

8. Koike T, Yamato Y, Yoshiya K, et al. Intentional limited pulmonary resection for peripheral T1 N0 M0 small-sized lung cancer. J Thorac Cardiovasc Surg 2003;125:924–8.

9. Landreneau RJ, Sugarbaker DJ, Mack MJ, et al. Wedge resection versus lobectomy for stage I (T1 N0 M0) non-small-cell lung cancer. J Thorac Cardiovasc Surg 1997;113:691–8 [discussion: 698–700].

10. Martin-Ucar AE, Nakas A, Pilling JE, et al. A case-matched study of anatomical segmentectomy versus lobectomy for stage I lung cancer in high-risk patients. Eur J Cardiothorac Surg 2005;27:675–9.

11. Okada M, Koike T, Higashiyama M, et al. Radical sublobar resection for small-sized non-small cell lung cancer: a multicenter study. J Thorac Cardiovasc Surg 2006;132:769–75.

12. Schuchert MJ, Pettiford BL, Keeley S, et al. Anatomic segmentectomy in the treatment of stage I non-small cell lung cancer. Ann Thorac Surg 2007; 84:926–32 [discussion: 932–3].

13. Bando T, Yamagihara K, Ohtake Y, et al. A new method of segmental resection for primary lung cancer: intermediate results. Eur J Cardiothorac Surg 2002;21:894–9 [discussion: 900].

14. Okada M, Nishio W, Sakamoto T, et al. Effect of tumor size on prognosis in patients with non-small cell lung cancer: the role of segmentectomy as a type of lesser resection. J Thorac Cardiovasc Surg 2005;129:87–93.

15. El-Sherif A, Fernando HC, Santos R, et al. Margin and local recurrence after sublobar resection of non-small cell lung cancer. Ann Surg Oncol 2007; 14:2400–5.

16. Kilic A, Schuchert MJ, Pettiford BL, et al. Anatomic segmentectomy for stage I non-small cell lung cancer in the elderly. Ann Thorac Surg 2009;87: 1662–6 [discussion: 7–8].

17. Sawabata N, Ohta M, Matsumura A, et al. Optimal distance of malignant negative margin in excision of nonsmall cell lung cancer: a multicenter prospective study. Ann Thorac Surg 2004;77:415–20.

18. Iwasaki A, Hamanaka W, Hamada T, et al. Comparison between a case-matched analysis of left upper lobe trisegmentectomy and left upper lobectomy for small size lung cancer located in the upper division. Thorac Cardiovasc Surg 2007;55(7):454–7.

19. Fernando HC, Santos RS, Benfield JR, et al. Lobar and sublobar resection with and without brachytherapy for small stage IA non-small cell lung cancer. J Thorac Cardiovasc Surg 2005;129:261–7.

20. Rami-Porta R, Ball D, Crowley J, et al. The IASLC Lung Cancer Staging Project: proposals for the revision of the T descriptors in the forthcoming (seventh) edition of the TNM classification for lung cancer. J Thorac Oncol 2007;2:593–602.

21. Naunheim KS, Kesler KA, D'Orazio SA, et al. Lung cancer surgery in the octogenarian. Eur J Cardiothorac Surg 1994;8(9):453–6.

22. Mery CM, Pappas AN, Bueno R, et al. Similar long-term survival of elderly patients with non-small cell lung cancer treated with lobectomy or wedge resection within the surveillance, epidemiology, and end results database. Chest 2005;128:237–45.

23. d'Amato TA, Galloway M, Szydlowski G, et al. Intraoperative brachytherapy following thoracoscopic wedge resection of stage I lung cancer. Chest 1998;114:1112–5.

24. Shennib H, Bogart J, Herndon JE, et al. Video-assisted wedge resection and local radiotherapy for peripheral lung cancer in high-risk patients: the Cancer and Leukemia Group B (CALGB) 9335, a phase II, multi-institutional cooperative group study. J Thorac Cardiovasc Surg 2005; 129:813–8.

25. Birdas TJ, Koehler RP, Colonias A, et al. Sublobar resection with brachytherapy versus lobectomy for stage Ib nonsmall cell lung cancer. Ann Thorac Surg 2006;81:434–8 [discussion: 8–9].

26. Lee W, Daly BD, DiPetrillo TA, et al. Limited resection for non-small cell lung cancer: observed local control with implantation of I-125 brachytherapy seeds. Ann Thorac Surg 2003;75:237–42 [discussion: 42–3].

27. Santos R, Colonias A, Parda D, et al. Comparison between sublobar resection and 125iodine brachytherapy after sublobar resection in high-risk patients with stage I non-small-cell lung cancer. Surgery 2003;134:691–7 [discussion: 697].

28. Fernando H, Landreneau R, Madnrekar S, et al. The impact of adjuvant brachytherapy with sublobar resection on pulmonary function and dyspnea: preliminary results from ACOSOG Z4032 trial. In: 90th Annual Meeting of the American Association for Thoracic Surgery. Toronto, Canada, 2010. p. 180.

29. Hiran C, Fernando RJ, Mandrekar SJ, et al. Thirty and ninety day outcomes after sublobar resection

for non-small cell lung cancer (NSCLC); results from a multicenter phase III study. Philadelphia: American Association for Thoracic Surgery; 2011.

30. McGarry RC, Song G, des Rosiers P, et al. Observation-only management of early stage, medically inoperable lung cancer: poor outcome. Chest 2002;121:1155–8.

31. Raz DJ, Zell JA, Ou SH, et al. Natural history of stage I non-small cell lung cancer: implications for early detection. Chest 2007;132:193–9.

32. Wisnivesky JP, Bonomi M, Henschke C, et al. Radiation therapy for the treatment of unresected stage I-II non-small cell lung cancer. Chest 2005;128:1461–7.

33. Qiao X, Tullgren O, Lax I, et al. The role of radiotherapy in treatment of stage I non-small cell lung cancer. Lung Cancer 2003;41:1–11.

34. Bogart JA, Hodgson L, Seagren SL, et al. Phase I study of accelerated conformal radiotherapy for stage I non-small-cell lung cancer in patients with pulmonary dysfunction: CALGB 39904. J Clin Oncol 2010;28:202–6.

35. Chen M, Hayman JA, Ten Haken RK, et al. Long-term results of high-dose conformal radiotherapy for patients with medically inoperable T1-3N0 non-small-cell lung cancer: is low incidence of regional failure due to incidental nodal irradiation? Int J Radiat Oncol Biol Phys 2006;64:120–6.

36. Fang LC, Komaki R, Allen P, et al. Comparison of outcomes for patients with medically inoperable stage I non-small-cell lung cancer treated with two-dimensional vs. three-dimensional radiotherapy. Int J Radiat Oncol Biol Phys 2006;66:108–16.

37. Blomgren H, Lax I, Naslund I, et al. Stereotactic high dose fraction radiation therapy of extracranial tumors using an accelerator. Clinical experience of the first thirty-one patients. Acta Oncol 1995;34:861–70.

38. Alam N, Flores RM. Video-assisted thoracic surgery (VATS) lobectomy: the evidence base. JSLS 2007;11:368–74.

39. Baumann P, Nyman J, Hoyer M, et al. Outcome in a prospective phase II trial of medically inoperable stage I non-small-cell lung cancer patients treated with stereotactic body radiotherapy. J Clin Oncol 2009;27:3290–6.

40. Collins BT, Erickson K, Reichner CA, et al. Radical stereotactic radiosurgery with real-time tumor motion tracking in the treatment of small peripheral lung tumors. Radiat Oncol 2007;2:39.

41. Fakiris AJ, McGarry RC, Yiannoutsos CT, et al. Stereotactic body radiation therapy for early-stage non-small-cell lung carcinoma: four-year results of a prospective phase II study. Int J Radiat Oncol Biol Phys 2009;75:677–82.

42. Fukumoto S, Shirato H, Shimzu S, et al. Small-volume image-guided radiotherapy using hypofractionated, coplanar, and noncoplanar multiple fields for patients with inoperable stage I nonsmall cell lung carcinomas. Cancer 2002;95:1546–53.

43. Koto M, Takai Y, Ogawa Y, et al. A phase II study on stereotactic body radiotherapy for stage I non-small cell lung cancer. Radiother Oncol 2007;85:429–34.

44. Le QT, Loo BW, Ho A, et al. Results of a phase I dose-escalation study using single-fraction stereotactic radiotherapy for lung tumors. J Thorac Oncol 2006;1:802–9.

45. Matsuo Y, Shibuya K, Nagata Y, et al. Prognostic factors in stereotactic body radiotherapy for non-small-cell lung cancer. Int J Radiat Oncol Biol Phys 2011;79(4):1104–11.

46. McGarry RC, Papiez L, Williams M, et al. Stereotactic body radiation therapy of early-stage non-small-cell lung carcinoma: phase I study. Int J Radiat Oncol Biol Phys 2005;63:1010–5.

47. Onimaru R, Fujino M, Yamazaki K, et al. Steep dose-response relationship for stage I non-small-cell lung cancer using hypofractionated high-dose irradiation by real-time tumor-tracking radiotherapy. Int J Radiat Oncol Biol Phys 2008;70:374–81.

48. Onishi H, Kuriyama K, Komiyama T, et al. Clinical outcomes of stereotactic radiotherapy for stage I non-small cell lung cancer using a novel irradiation technique: patient self-controlled breath-hold and beam switching using a combination of linear accelerator and CT scanner. Lung Cancer 2004;45:45–55.

49. Ricardi U, Filippi AR, Guarneri A, et al. Stereotactic body radiation therapy for early stage non-small cell lung cancer: results of a prospective trial. Lung Cancer 2010;68:72–7.

50. Timmerman R, Paulus R, Galvin J, et al. Stereotactic body radiation therapy for inoperable early stage lung cancer. JAMA 2010;303:1070–6.

51. Xia T, Li H, Sun Q, et al. Promising clinical outcome of stereotactic body radiation therapy for patients with inoperable stage I/II non-small-cell lung cancer. Int J Radiat Oncol Biol Phys 2006;66:117–25.

52. Yoon SM, Choi EK, Lee SW, et al. Clinical results of stereotactic body frame based fractionated radiation therapy for primary or metastatic thoracic tumors. Acta Oncol 2006;45:1108–14.

53. Grutters JP, Kessels AG, Pijls-Johannesma M, et al. Comparison of the effectiveness of radiotherapy with photons, protons and carbon-ions for non-small cell lung cancer: a meta-analysis. Radiother Oncol 2010;95:32–40.

54. Henderson M, McGarry R, Yiannoutsos C, et al. Baseline pulmonary function as a predictor for survival and decline in pulmonary function over time in patients undergoing stereotactic body radiotherapy for the treatment of stage I non-small-cell lung cancer. Int J Radiat Oncol Biol Phys 2008;72:404–9.

55. Timmerman R, McGarry R, Yiannoutsos C, et al. Excessive toxicity when treating central tumors in a phase II study of stereotactic body radiation

therapy for medically inoperable early-stage lung cancer. J Clin Oncol 2006;24:4833–9.

56. Beland MD, Wasser EJ, Mayo-Smith WW, et al. Primary non-small cell lung cancer: review of frequency, location, and time of recurrence after radiofrequency ablation. Radiology 2010;254:301–7.

57. Fernando HC, De Hoyos A, Landreneau RJ, et al. Radiofrequency ablation for the treatment of non-small cell lung cancer in marginal surgical candidates. J Thorac Cardiovasc Surg 2005;129:639–44.

58. Grieco CA, Simon CJ, Mayo-Smith WW, et al. Percutaneous image-guided thermal ablation and radiation therapy: outcomes of combined treatment for 41 patients with inoperable stage I/II non-small-cell lung cancer. J Vasc Interv Radiol 2006;17:1117–24.

59. Hsie M, Morbidini-Gaffney S, Kohman LJ, et al. Definitive treatment of poor-risk patients with stage I lung cancer: a single institution experience. J Thorac Oncol 2009;4:69–73.

60. Lanuti M, Sharma A, Digumarthy SR, et al. Radiofrequency ablation for treatment of medically inoperable stage I non-small cell lung cancer. J Thorac Cardiovasc Surg 2009;137:160–6.

61. Lee JM, Jin GY, Goldberg SN, et al. Percutaneous radiofrequency ablation for inoperable non-small cell lung cancer and metastases: preliminary report. Radiology 2004;230:125–34.

62. Lencioni R, Crocetti L, Cioni R, et al. Response to radiofrequency ablation of pulmonary tumours: a prospective, intention-to-treat, multicentre clinical trial (the RAPTURE study). Lancet Oncol 2008;9: 621–8.

63. Pennathur A, Luketich JD, Abbas G, et al. Radiofrequency ablation for the treatment of stage I non-small cell lung cancer in high-risk patients. J Thorac Cardiovasc Surg 2007;134:857–64.

64. Simon CJ, Dupuy DE, DiPetrillo TA, et al. Pulmonary radiofrequency ablation: long-term safety and efficacy in 153 patients. Radiology 2007;243:268–75.

65. Gomez FM, Palussiere J, Santos E, et al. Radiofrequency thermocoagulation of lung tumours. Where we are, where we are headed. Clin Transl Oncol 2009;11:28–34.

66. Belfiore G, Moggio G, Tedeschi E, et al. CT-guided radiofrequency ablation: a potential complementary therapy for patients with unresectable primary lung cancer–a preliminary report of 33 patients. AJR Am J Roentgenol 2004;183:1003–11.

67. Dupuy DE, DiPetrillo T, Gandhi S, et al. Radiofrequency ablation followed by conventional radiotherapy for medically inoperable stage I non-small cell lung cancer. Chest 2006;129:738–45.

68. Hiraki T, Gobara H, Iishi T, et al. Percutaneous radiofrequency ablation for clinical stage I non-small cell lung cancer: results in 20 nonsurgical candidates. J Thorac Cardiovasc Surg 2007;134:1306–12.

69. Nachiappan AC, Sharma A, Shepard JA, et al. Radiofrequency ablation in the lung complicated by positive airway pressure ventilation. Ann Thorac Surg 2010;89:1665–7.

70. Zhu JC, Yan TD, Glenn D, et al. Radiofrequency ablation of lung tumors: feasibility and safety. Ann Thorac Surg 2009;87:1023–8.

71. Sano Y, Kanazawa S, Gobara H, et al. Feasibility of percutaneous radiofrequency ablation for intrathoracic malignancies: a large single-center experience. Cancer 2007;109:1397–405.

72. de Baere T, Palussiere J, Auperin A, et al. Midterm local efficacy and survival after radiofrequency ablation of lung tumors with minimum follow-up of 1 year: prospective evaluation. Radiology 2006;240: 587–96.

73. Ali MK, Mountain CF, Ewer MS, et al. Predicting loss of pulmonary function after pulmonary resection for bronchogenic carcinoma. Chest 1980;77(3):337–42.

74. Yoo D, Dupuy DE, Hillman S. Radiofrequency ablation of medically inoperable stage IA non-small cell lung cancer: are early posttreatment PET findings predictive of treatment outcome? Am J Roentol 2011;197(2):334–40.

75. Wang H, Littrup PJ, Duan Y, et al. Thoracic masses treated with percutaneous cryotherapy: initial experience with more than 200 procedures. Radiology 2005;235:289–98.

76. Wolf FJ, Grand DJ, Machan JT, et al. Microwave ablation of lung malignancies: effectiveness, CT findings, and safety in 50 patients. Radiology 2008;247:871–9.

77. Thurer RJ. Cryotherapy in early lung cancer. Chest 2001;120:3–5.

Induction Therapy for Lung Cancer: Sailing Across the Pillars of Hercules

Gaetano Rocco, MD, FRCSEd[a],*, Alessandro Morabito, MD[b],
Paolo Muto, MD[c]

KEYWORDS

- Lung cancer • Induction therapy • Neoadjuvant treatment
- Locally advanced non–small cell lung cancer

In 2011, physicians pursuing an integrated care for lung cancer patients have finally moved away from separate treatment compartments. Indeed, there have been times when the only concern among clinicians was to assess whether lung cancer was deemed resectable or not. The range of tumor resectability was unknown to the surgeons themselves who had only chest radiographs and stratigrams to rely on at a time when exploratory thoracotomy seemed to be the final diagnostic tool. At what price for the patient was not deemed to be a deciding factor. The concept of operability referred to a rudimentary assessment of the cardiorespiratory and medical condition finalized to determine surgical eligibility. It was the era of treatment-centered management when patients were subjected to chest radiographs and taken straight to theater for rigid bronchoscopy to confirm that the endoscopic extent of the tumor would be compatible with the anticipated anatomic resection. Standard, muscle-dividing, thoracotomy and a very low threshold for removing the entire lung were common. The Lung Cancer Study Group trial[1] and the reintroduction of video-assisted thoracoscopic surgery have modernized General Thoracic Surgery by focusing on patient-centered, minimally invasive, parenchyma-saving pulmonary resections.

With the introduction into clinical practice of computed tomography (CT) scanning and refined staging systems, the concept of locally advanced disease became established. Two milestone articles have led the way in the implementation of neoadjuvant or induction treatment in lung cancer management.[2,3] In spite of numerous clinical trials the jury is still out on the value of induction therapy for locally advanced lung cancer.[4] The authors elected to address this topic from the multifaceted views of the clinicians often involved in lung cancer management and according to the most recent views on the concept of locally advanced non–small cell lung cancer (NSCLC)[4–8] (European Society for Medical Oncology [ESMO]; National Institute of Clinical Excellence [NICE] guidelines; American College of Chest Physicians; National Comprehensive Cancer Network [NCCN]; British Thoracic Society). Recently, the International Association for the Study of Lung Cancer Lung Cancer Study Group has validated the concept of a prognostic stratification of N2 disease subsets, especially single-zone versus multiple-zone N2.[8,9] On the verge of such substantial

[a] Lung Cancer Multidisciplinary Team, Division of Thoracic Surgery, Department of Thoracic Surgery and Oncology, National Cancer Institute, Pascale Foundation, Naples, Italy
[b] Lung Cancer Multidisciplinary Team, Division of Medical Oncology, Department of Thoracic Surgery and Oncology, National Cancer Institute, Pascale Foundation, Naples, Italy
[c] Lung Cancer Multidisciplinary Team, Division of Radiation Oncology, National Cancer Institute, Pascale Foundation, Naples, Italy
* Corresponding author. Division of Thoracic Surgery, Department of Thoracic Surgery and Oncology, National Cancer Institute, Pascale Foundation, Via Semmola, 80131, Naples, Italy.
E-mail address: Gaetano.Rocco@btopenworld.com

Thorac Surg Clin 22 (2012) 67–75
doi:10.1016/j.thorsurg.2011.08.010
1547-4127/12/$ – see front matter © 2012 Elsevier Inc. All rights reserved.

changes being implemented in the interpretation of locally advanced NSCLC, 10 crucial issues were identified, which may have an impact on the approach to patients with locally advanced lung cancer in everyday practice.

A DECALOGUE ON INDUCTION TREATMENT IN 2011

A rigid, scholastic approach to locally advanced NSCLC is far from the practical management philosophy shared by the majority of surgeons.[10] Much has been said and done. However, a few controversial issues in the surgical practice need to be clarified in the attempt to define a user-friendly decalogue for surgeons practicing in 2011.

Neoadjuvant Treatment Serves the Purpose of Converting a Nonresectable into a Resectable Tumor

Several potential advantages of induction chemotherapy for NSCLC are known to clinicians, including the possible downstaging of the disease, the evaluation on surgical specimens of the efficacy of chemotherapeutic agents, the likelihood to control asymptomatic metastases and reduce the surgery-related cancerous dissemination.[8] However, the reported resection rate after induction treatment may vary considerably.[11] Sixteen series of trimodality treatment were analyzed by Kunitoh and Suzuki,[11] who noted that in 5 of them no resection rate was available. The remaining 11 series reported resection rates ranging between 43% and 93%.[11] Of interest, the larger-numbered series resulting from retrospective studies either had no specification of the resection rate or, if it had, the figure ranged between 50% and 60%.[11] The best resection rates were seen for a total number of surgical cases slightly in excess of 100 surgical patients.[11] With the exception of superior sulcus tumors, patients with locally advanced lung cancer should not be subjected to induction treatment with the aim of improving resectability.[11] Absence of progression or partial response to chemotherapy or chemoradiotherapy on the coexisting diseased nodes represents grounds enough to improve oncologic operability (ie, downstaging to N0–1).[7,8]

The Presence of Mediastinal Nodal Disease Ipsilateral to the T (ie, N2) is a Relative Contraindication to Surgical Resection as Primary Treatment Modality

Consensus emerges from the surgical literature about the existence of different subsets of N2 disease, each portending a specific prognostic outlook (**Table 1**).[4,6,8,9,12] In fact, an important distinction is to be made between N2 detected before thoracotomy/video-assisted thoracoscopic surgery (VATS) and subsequent pulmonary resection and N2 found at the time of surgery. Ferguson[13] has rigorously demonstrated the increasing costs and the uncertain benefits resulting from performing pulmonary resection when intraoperative N2 disease is diagnosed. However, the vast majority of surgeons would treat intraoperatively found, single-station N2, especially on the left side, as a subset with acceptable 5-year survival rates.[10,14] In 2011, the NICE issued the revised guidelines (previously published in 2005) on lung cancer management, contemplating the possibility to primarily resect single-station N2 and emphasizing the need for surgery-centered trials to address the role of surgery.[5] The paradigm shift is obvious inasmuch as it is suggested to move away from the concept of surgery as a detrimental factor in multimodality treatment strategies because of its morbidity/mortality rates, especially if pneumonectomy was necessary.[5] Indeed, apart from surgery not being harmful to patients after neoadjuvant regimens, another aspect of the NICE guidelines needs consideration, namely that certain N2 subsets (ie, single-zone N2) may "intuitively" benefit from surgery.[5] The recently published British Thoracic Society guidelines apparently make a step forward by recommending surgery for single-zone N2 disease also outside the context of clinical trials, which continue to be advised for N2 multizone and N3 disease.[8] Be that as it may, NCCN institutions make a strong point in aggressively defining the pathologic nature of mediastinal nodal disease prior to outlining a management protocol for the individual patient with locally advanced NSCLC.[7] The idea of proceeding to primary surgery even for single-zone disease without prior histologic characterization is not accepted (**Table 2**).[7]

T4 N0 Could Benefit from Primary Surgery but it is a Relatively Rare Presentation of NSCLC

As a consequence, the accumulation of considerable experience in resecting this challenging tumor subset may be difficult.[8] Indeed, only a few surgical centers have reported on extended resections to mediastinal vascular structures, the carina, esophagus, or the vertebrae; almost invariably, the series include few tens of patients with about 5 procedures for the specific T4 subgroup performed per year.[8,15–19] The reported 5-year survival after surgery for T4 lung cancer can be as high as 38%, with acceptable mortality rates (4%).[16] The need for minimally invasive surgical

Table 1
The European view on the management of stage IIIA NSCLC

NSCLC N2 Subset[4]	Surgery Primary	Induction	Additional Chemotherapy/ Radiotherapy	Primary Chemotherapy	Primary Radiotherapy	Surgery Post Induction
N2 at final pathology (IIIA-1)	Yes	—	Yes	—	—	—
Occult (IIIA-2)	Yes	—	Yes	—	—	—
Preoperative single (IIIA-3) zone	Yes	Not	Yes	Yes if inoperable	Yes if inoperable	—
Preoperative left-sided station 5 IIIA-3	Yes	—	Yes	Yes if inoperable	Yes if inoperable	—
Preoperative right-sided upper lobe and single N2 Barety	Yes	—	Yes	—	—	—
Preoperative multiple (IIIA-3)	Not	Yes	—	Yes	Not	If CR/PR
Preoperative subcarinal (IIIA-3)	Yes?	—	Yes	Yes	?	If CR/PR
Postinduction CR	—	—	—	Yes	—	Yes
Postinduction persistent	—	—	?	Yes	?	Yes if PR >50%
Postinduction surgery recalcitrant	—	—	Yes	Yes	?	—

Abbreviations: CR, complete remission; PR, partial remission.

Table 2
The North American view on the management of stage IIIA NSCLC

NSCLC N2 Subset[4]	Primary Surgery	Induction	Additional Chemotherapy/ Radiotherapy	Primary Chemotherapy Definitive	Primary Radiotherapy Definitive	Surgery Post Induction
N2 at final pathology (IIIA-1)	Yes	—	Yes	—	—	—
Occult (IIIA-2)	Yes	—	Yes	—	—	—
Preoperative single[a] (IIIA-3) zone	Not	Yes	Yes if inoperable	Yes if inoperable	Yes if inoperable	Yes
Preoperative left-sided station 5 IIIA-3	Not	Yes	Yes if inoperable	Yes if inoperable	Yes if inoperable	Yes
Preoperative right-sided upper lobe and single N2 Barety	Not	Yes	Yes if inoperable	Yes if inoperable	Yes if inoperable	Yes
Preoperative multiple (IIIA-3)	Not	Yes	Yes	Yes	Yes	If no progression
Preoperative subcarinal (IIIA-3)	Not	Yes	Yes	Yes	?	If no progression
Postinduction CR	—	—	—	Yes	—	Yes
Postinduction persistent	—	—	?	Yes	?	Yes if PR >50%
Postinduction surgery recalcitrant	—	—	Yes	Yes	?	—

[a] <3 cm.

exploration (ie, by VATS) of the chest before denying the cT4 patient a surgical option has been suggested by several investigators during the years.[20,21] Equally emphasized is the dismal prognosis entailed by primary surgery for T4N2.[22] Such clinical findings have indicated trial designs of induction chemotherapy that separated T4N0-1 from N2 disease.[23] In this study from Spain on 139 patients all receiving at least one cycle of cisplatin-gemcitabine-docetaxel prior to surgery, similar 5-year survival rates were observed in both N2 and T4N0-1 groups.[23] Confirming prevailing views in this field, complete resection after induction therapy, yielding an intriguing 41% 5-year survival, was a significant predictor of long-term survival on multivariate analysis along with clinical response and age younger than 60 years.[23] The ESMO guidelines include the T4N0-1 among locally advanced NSCLC subsets amenable to resection and adjuvant treatment (IIIA 0–2).[4] General consensus exists on the need for careful selection of patients with stage IIIB disease to be entered into clinical trials of multimodality treatment.[8]

Superior Sulcus Tumors: A T4 of its Own

With the refinement of surgical techniques and the advancement of induction regimens, the management of superior sulcus tumors has evolved in time to include subsequent treatment paradigms focused on radiotherapy alone, induction radiotherapy plus surgery, and chemoradiotherapy followed by resection.[24,25] Conventional radiotherapy (45–70 Gy) reportedly failed to achieve consistently satisfactory 5-year survivals (6%)[24] whereas pain control is achieved in more than 75% of the patients.[24] Nowadays, 3-dimensional conformal radiotherapy (3D-CT) or intensity-modulated radiation treatment (IMRT) are used to synchronize the administration of radiotherapy with the respiratory cycle ("gating"), precisely deliver higher volumes to the target lesion, and at the same time avoid toxicity to neurovascular structures at the thoracic inlet.[26] Conversely, induction radiotherapy (30 Gy) and surgery have been shown to yield R0 resection rates and overall 5-year survivals of 50% and 30%, respectively.[24,27] Trimodality regimens (including radiotherapy schedules up to 45–60 Gy[26]) have contributed to completeness of resection, with 5-year survivals reported to range between 68% and 100% (mean, 87%) and between 40% and 84%, (mean, 55%), respectively.[24] Consensus seems to exist on the favorable impact on prognosis after complete surgical resection including at least a lobectomy in the absence of mediastinal

ipsilateral or contralateral nodal disease.[24,27] As for other T4 subsets, the availability of specific surgical approaches and techniques to the thoracic inlet has allowed criteria for resectability to be extended to vascular, vertebral, and localized neural (brachial plexus) infiltration by superior sulcus neoplasms.[24] As a consequence, local control rates after trimodality induction regimens are in excess of 70% and may reach 100%.[24,28] In fact, Marra and colleagues[29] recently reported a 6.4% rate of local recurrences (2 patients of 31 with T3/T4 Pancoast tumors treated with induction chemotherapy followed by chemoradiotherapy and surgery in selected cases) combined in one patient with distant relapse. In this context, brain metastases represent a frequent site of distant relapse (up to 40% in the Intergroup Trial [INT] 0160[30]) and pose the need for prophylactic brain irradiation following the pulmonary resection.[26,29]

Positron Emission Tomography, the Introduction of VATS and Endobronchial Ultrasonography in the Staging of NSCLC, and the Reduction of Exploratory Thoracotomies

The latter should be on rare occasions reserved to assess resectability (ie, the T compartment) and not to confirm operability (N2 vs N3).[8] In this context, positron emission tomography (PET)/CT is used to guide the need for histologic verification.[31] Although consensus seems to exist as to mediastinal exploration to confirm PET-positive N2/3, PET-negative nodes may hide metastatic disease in 1 out of 5 and would still support the resort to mediastinoscopy.[31,32] In the latter scenario, endobronchial ultrasonography (EBUS), for which the instrumentation and the necessary expertise are both available, is replacing mediastinoscopy in the primary staging modality of the mediastinum by virtue of sensitivity and specificity of 93% and 100%, respectively.[8] One often forgotten but distinct advantage of the endoscopic ultrasound-guided approach is the potential to biopsy the left adrenal gland and the left lobe of the liver.[8] However, mediastinoscopy is still considered the gold standard for mediastinal staging.[8] If EBUS is used for staging and the patient receives induction treatment, mediastinoscopy can be used to restage the mediastinum to appropriately select N2 patients for surgery.[33] If mediastinoscopy is chosen to primarily stage the mediastinum, the negative predictive value of EBUS at restaging can be as low as 20%.[34] In specific circumstances, VATS can be also used to sample or remove mediastinal nodes according to the principles of minimal invasiveness.[8] More recently, proponents of prethoracotomy extensive nodal dissection either through video-assisted mediastinoscopic lymphadenectomy (VAMLA) or total mediastinoscopic lymphadenectomy (TEMLA) have made the case for a routine bilateral removal of accessible nodal stations (including 5L and 6L) to improve patient selection for surgery.[35,36] When TEMLA was used to confirm EBUS results at restaging after induction treatment, the negative predictive value of EBUS increased to 67%.[37]

Technical Issues After Induction Treatment

Whether resection after neoadjuvant therapy should encompass the disease extent, the original T or the T assessed at restaging is not clear.[38] Current literature reports the resort to pneumonectomy after induction treatment for anywhere between 20% and 40% of the patients.[11,39] Weder and colleagues[39] reported on a particularly significant series because chemoradiotherapy regimens were used in 80% of the patients; an obvious interpretation is that, despite maximum effort at achieving local control, surgical resection had to encompass the entire lung in the vast majority of these patients. This finding is relevant if one takes into consideration the prevalence of stage IIB and IIIA (45% of the total pneumonectomies performed[39]). In such circumstances, chemoradiotherapy may make lymph nodes tightly adhere to the adventitia of the hilar vessels ("frozen hilum").[11] Experienced surgeons will frequently secure the main pulmonary vessels proximally, as a rule within the pericardium, before attempting nodal dissection.[11] How far this dissection needs to be performed in the face of risking potentially catastrophic hemorrhages depends on several factors. Nevertheless, the concept of balancing the effort aiming at a complete nodal dissection against the risk for major intraoperative blood loss must be carefully evaluated by the surgeon.[11,40]

One of the recurrent nightmares surfacing in the thoracic surgeons' collective unconscious is the onset of bronchopleural fistula (BPF) after pulmonary resection.[11] Trimodality regimens reportedly have been plagued with BPF rates up to 15% despite prophylactic bronchial stump coverage.[11] Moreover, induction treatment may expose patients to postresection pulmonary edema which, in turn, may be responsible for the development of acute respiratory distress syndrome. Careful fluid balance should be maintained in the postoperative course of these patients to avoid interstitial extravasation, especially after pneumonectomy. The quality of the surgical approach tends to be homogeneously safe in reports from individual institutions rather than in multicentric studies.[11,41] One of the possible pitfalls in the design of a randomized controlled trial (RCT) of induction treatment for locally advanced NSCLC resides in the heterogeneity of surgery with regard to the use of parenchyma-saving resections, and the extent of nodal dissection.[38]

Induction Chemoradiation Carries Different Morbidity and Mortality Rates Compared with Induction Chemotherapy Alone

Primary resection for lung cancer entails mortality rates ranging from 1.3% to 3.7%,[42] namely 1.2% to 2.9% and 3.2% to 6.2% for lobectomy and pneumonectomy, respectively. Following induction treatment, the percentages increase to 2.4% to 3.8% for lobectomy and 7.2% to 12% for pneumonectomy.[42] All in all, the surgical literature tends not to consider resection after induction chemotherapy at a substantially increased operative risks.[41,43] However, the addition of radiotherapy in a trimodality neoadjuvant regimen is reported to carry a 10% treatment-related mortality rate.[11] Nevertheless, Weder and colleagues[39] have recently demonstrated the safety of pneumonectomy after induction treatment by reporting a 3% mortality rate and a 38% 5-year survival rate from a bi-institutional study including 176 patients.

Local Control and Complete Response After Neoadjuvant Treatment: Lessons Learned from EORTC 08941 and INT 0139

Crinò and colleagues[4] have made interesting observations regarding two recently conducted trials of induction treatment for locally advanced lung cancer, European Organization for the Research and Treatment of Cancer (EORTC) 08941 and INT 0139. In the former, patients were subjected to induction platinum–based chemotherapy and then randomly allocated to either surgery or radiotherapy (up to 60 Gy).[44] Conversely, in INT 0139 the two treatment arms consisted of induction chemoradiotherapy (cisplatin and etoposide; 45 Gy) followed by surgery compared with chemoradiotherapy (same regimen with radiotherapy increasing up to 61 Gy) only.[45] In addition to overlapping results in terms overall survival between surgery and radiation treatment, the potential for pathologic downstaging demonstrated by both induction regimens was low (approximately 40%).[4] Another worrisome detail is the reduced discriminating ability of persistent N2 for current imaging technology.[4] Both trials confirmed that surgery remains the best modality to achieve local control, especially in downstaged patients subjected to lobectomy.[4,38] Concerns about the impact of morbidity and mortality after pneumonectomy are clearly voiced in the two trials.[44,45] As already noted, recent evidence provided from authoritative surgical centers seems to dispute these findings.[39]

Neoadjuvant Treatment Regimens for Stage III NSCLC

Neoadjuvant chemotherapy has become a recommended treatment for potentially resectable stage IIIA-N2 NSCLC.[46,47] In the early 1990s, two small randomized phase 3 trials had demonstrated an advantage in survival of induction chemotherapy with second-generation platinum combinations followed by surgery versus surgery alone.[2,3] Subsequent clinical studies and meta-analyses have increased the evidence of the activity as well as the good tolerability of this approach.[48–50] In the aforementioned EORTC 08941 trial, the induction chemotherapy consisted of 3 cycles of cisplatin, at a dose of at least 80 mg/m^2 per cycle, or carboplatin, at a target area under the curve of at least 5 per cycle, combined with at least one other chemotherapy drug (mainly gemcitabine or taxanes).[44] In the INT 0139 trial,[45] the induction chemotherapy was 2 cycles of cisplatin (50 mg/m^2 on days 1, 8, 29, and 36, intravenous infusions) and etoposide (50 mg/m^2 on days 1–5 and 29–33, intravenous infusions), administered in combination with induction thoracic radiotherapy (45 Gy) beginning on day 1, in 1.8-Gy daily fractions. Therefore, with the present status of knowledge, preoperative platinum-based combination chemotherapy can be considered in patients with stage IIIA-N2 disease: a 2-drug combination of platinum and a third-generation drug seems preferable and at least 3 cycles of chemotherapy should be administered. As to radiotherapy for N3 disease, a total dose of 60 to 66 Gy is delivered on PET-positive mediastinal and supraclavicular nodal stations along with the T compartment. To avoid or reduce the likelihood of significant pulmonary toxicity when treating Pancoast tumors, the authors use constraint doses of hyperfractionated 3D-CT with an MLD <20 Gy; V20 (volume of lung receiving 20 Gy) <30%; V25 <25%; and V30 <15%. In addition, neighboring structures are protected by V50 <30% (esophagus); V50 <40% (heart); and maximal doses of 60 Gy and 50 Gy for the brachial plexus and the spine, respectively.

Interpretation of Meta-Analysis and Recommendations for Everyday Practice

A thoracic surgeon, questioned by his or her patient on providing figures summarizing the advantages of induction treatment, should provide a realistic answer based on the available literature. Neoadjuvant therapy may entail a 6% to 7%

survival benefit for patients with clinical IIIA, thereby prospecting 5-year survival rate ranging between 21% and 42%.[4,47,51] On the other hand, RCT results are difficult to interpret. As demonstrated by the most studied EORTC 08941 and INT 0139,[44,45] apart from the lack of substantial data for the specific stage III subsets and the attendant survival stratification, low numerosity and heterogeneous surgical approach in the surgical arms along with the uncertain administration of adjuvant therapy make available data from currently available trials of induction treatment simply a "best guess."[10,38] The most recent guidelines from Europe seem to indicate that primary surgery may be recommended for selected patients with T4N0-1 and nonbulky, single-zone N2 disease.[5,8] In this setting, Pancoast tumors may benefit from induction chemoradiotherapy aimed at increasing local control.[30,52] In 2011, these can be acknowledged as the Pillars of Hercules of induction treatment for lung cancer. Beyond the Columns, there is a foggy open sea of randomized trials being prematurely closed because of incomplete accrual or failure to robustly demonstrate survival differences[53]; where the absolute ratio of maximum standardized uptake value in establishing metastatic nodal disease needs to be clarified[54]; where the jury is still out as to if and when, Pancoast excluded, preoperative chemotherapy should be used in lieu of induction chemoradiotherapy; and where a definitive pathway for mediastinal exploration for staging and restaging will be finally outlined. For now, all other stage III subsets should be offered multimodality management in the context of rigorously designed clinical trials.

REFERENCES

1. Ginsberg RJ, Rubinstein LV. Randomized trial of lobectomy versus limited resection for T1 N0 non-small cell lung cancer. Lung Cancer Study Group. Ann Thorac Surg 1995;60:615–23.
2. Rosell R, Gomez-Codina J, Camps C, et al. A randomized trial comparing preoperative chemotherapy plus surgery with surgery alone in patients with non-small-cell lung cancer. N Engl J Med 1994;330:153–8.
3. Roth JA, Fossella F, Komaki R, et al. A randomized trial comparing perioperative chemotherapy and surgery with surgery alone in resectable stage IIIA non-small-cell lung cancer. J Natl Cancer Inst 1994;86:673–80.
4. Crinò L, Weder W, van Meerbeeck J, et al, ESMO Guidelines Working Group. Early stage and locally advanced (non-metastatic) non-small-cell lung cancer: ESMO Clinical Practice Guidelines for

diagnosis, treatment and follow-up. Ann Oncol 2010; 21(Suppl 5):v103–15.

5. The National Institute of Clinical Excellence. Lung cancer: the diagnosis and treatment of lung cancer. 2011; Available at: http://www.nice.org.uk/guidance/CG121. Accessed September 7, 2011.

6. Robinson LA, Ruckdeschel JC, Wagner H, et al. Treatment of non-small cell lung cancer-stage IIIA: ACCP evidence-based clinical practice guidelines (2nd edition). Chest 2007;132(Suppl 3):243S–65S.

7. Ettinger DS, Akerley W, Bepler G, et al; NCCN Non-Small Cell Lung Cancer Panel Members. Non-small cell lung cancer. J Natl Compr Canc Netw 2010;8:740–801.

8. Lim E, Baldwin D, Beckles M, et al, British Thoracic Society, Society for Cardiothoracic Surgery in Great Britain and Ireland. Guidelines on the radical management of patients with lung cancer. Thorax 2010;65(Suppl 3):iii1–27.

9. Rusch VW, Crowley J, Giroux DJ, et al, International Staging Committee, Cancer Research and Biostatistics, Observers to the Committee, Participating Institutions. The IASLC Lung Cancer Staging Project: proposals for the revision of the N descriptors in the forthcoming seventh edition of the TNM classification for lung cancer. J Thorac Oncol 2007;2:603–12.

10. Rocco G. Results of cutting-edge surgery in stage IIIA-N2 nonsmall cell lung cancer. Curr Opin Oncol 2009;21:105–9.

11. Kunitoch H, Suzuki K. How to evaluate the risk/benefit of trimodality therapy in locally advanced non-small cell lung cancer. Br J Cancer 2007;96:1498–503.

12. Andre F, Grunenwald D, Pignon JP, et al. Survival of patients with resected N2 non-small-cell lung cancer: evidence for a subclassification and implications. J Clin Oncol 2000;18:2981–9.

13. Ferguson MK. Optimal management when unsuspected N2 nodal disease is identified during thoracotomy for lung cancer: cost-effectiveness analysis. J Thorac Cardiovasc Surg 2003;126:1935–42.

14. Detterbeck F. What to do with "surprise"N2? Intraoperative management of patients with non-small cell lung cancer. J Thorac Oncol 2008;3:289–302.

15. Daly BD, Ebright MI, Walkey AJ, et al. Impact of neoadjuvant chemoradiotherapy followed by surgical resection on node-negative T3 and T4 non-small cell lung cancer. J Thorac Cardiovasc Surg 2011;141:1392–7.

16. Yildizeli B, Dartevelle PG, Fadel E, et al. Results of primary surgery with T4 non-small cell lung cancer during a 25-year period in a single center: the benefit is worth the risk. Ann Thorac Surg 2008;86:1065–75.

17. Shargall Y, de Perrot M, Keshavjee S, et al. 15 years single center experience with surgical resection of the superior vena cava for non-small cell lung cancer. Lung Cancer 2004;45:357–63.

18. Ohta M, Hirabayasi H, Shiono H, et al. Surgical resection for lung cancer with infiltration of the thoracic aorta. J Thorac Cardiovasc Surg 2005; 129:804–8.

19. Mitchell JD, Mathisen DJ, Wright CD, et al. Resection for bronchogenic carcinoma involving the carina: long-term results and effect of nodal status on outcome. J Thorac Cardiovasc Surg 2001;121:465–71.

20. De Giacomo T, Rendina EA, Venuta F, et al. Thoracoscopic staging of IIIB non-small cell lung cancer before neoadjuvant therapy. Ann Thorac Surg 1997;64:1409–11.

21. Eggeling S, Martin T, Böttger J, et al. Invasive staging of non-small cell lung cancer—a prospective study. Eur J Cardiothorac Surg 2002;22:679–84.

22. Spaggiari L, Thomas P, Magdeleinat P, et al. Superior vena cava resection with prosthetic replacement for non-small cell lung cancer: long-term results of a multicentric study. Eur J Cardiothorac Surg 2002; 21:1080–6.

23. Garrido P, Gonzalez-Larriba JL, Insa A, et al. Long-term survival associated with complete resection after induction chemotherapy in stage IIIA (N2) and IIIB (T4N0-1) non small-cell lung cancer patients: the Spanish Lung Cancer Group Trial 9901. J Clin Oncol 2007;25:4736–42.

24. Tamura M, Hoda MA, Klepetko W. Current treatment paradigms of superior sulcus tumours. Eur J Cardiothorac Surg 2009;36:747–53.

25. Rusch VW. Management of Pancoast tumors. Lancet Oncol 2006;7:997–1005.

26. Kwong KF, Edelman MJ, Suntharalingam M, et al. High-dose radiotherapy in trimodality treatment of Pancoast tumors results in high pathologic complete response rates and excellent long-term survival. J Thorac Cardiovasc Surg 2005;129:1250–7.

27. Detterbeck FC, Jones DR, Rosenman JG. Pancoast tumors. In: Detterbeck FC, Rivera MP, Socinski MA, et al, editors. Diagnosis and treatment of lung cancer: an evidence-based guide for the practicing clinician. Philadelphia: WB Saunders; 2001. p. 233–43.

28. Wright G, Manser RL, Byrnes G, et al. Surgery for non-small cell lung cancer: systematic review and meta-analysis of randomised controlled trials. Thorax 2006;61:597–603.

29. Marra A, Eberhardt W, Pöttgen C, et al. Induction chemotherapy, concurrent chemoradiation and surgery for Pancoast tumour. Eur Respir J 2007;29:117–26.

30. Rusch VW, Giroux DJ, Kraut MJ, et al. Induction chemoradiation and surgical resection for non-small cell lung carcinomas of the superior sulcus: initial results of Southwest Oncology Group Trial 9416 (Intergroup Trial 0160). J Thorac Cardiovasc Surg 2001;121:472–83.

31. Woolley SM, Rajesh PB. The use of PET and PET/CT scanning in lung cancer. Asian Cardiovasc Thorac Ann 2008;16:353–4.

32. de Langen AJ, Raijmakers P, Riphagen I, et al. The size of mediastinal lymph nodes and its relation with metastatic involvement: a meta-analysis. Eur J Cardiothorac Surg 2006;29:26–9.

33. Pass HI. Lung cancer staging techniques and induction therapy: maybe timing is everything. J Clin Oncol 2008;26:3306–7.

34. Herth FJ, Annema JT, Yasufuku K, et al. Endobronchial ultrasound with transbronchial needle aspiration for restaging the mediastinum in lung cancer. J Clin Oncol 2008;26:3346–50.

35. Kuzdzal J, Zielinski M, Papla B, et al. The transcervical extended mediastinal lymphadenectomy versus cervical mediastinoscopy in non-small cell lung cancer staging. Eur J Cardiothorac Surg 2007;31: 88–94.

36. Witte B, Hürtgen M. Video-assisted mediastinoscopic lymphadenectomy (VAMLA). J Thorac Oncol 2007;2:367–9.

37. Szlubowski A, Herth FJ, Soja J, et al. Endobronchial ultrasound-guided needle aspiration in non-small-cell lung cancer restaging verified by the transcervical bilateral extended mediastinal lymphadenectomy— a prospective study. Eur J Cardiothorac Surg 2010; 37:1180–4.

38. Rocco G. Lobectomy after induction therapy for stage IIIA NSCLC in the presence of persistent N2 disease. In: Ferguson MK, editor. Difficult decisions in thoracic surgery, an evidence based approach. 2nd edition. London: Springer-Verlag; 2011. p. 111–7.

39. Weder W, Collaud S, Eberhardt WE, et al. Pneumonectomy is a valuable treatment option after neoadjuvant therapy for stage III non-small-cell lung cancer. J Thorac Cardiovasc Surg 2010;139: 1424–30.

40. Brichkov I, Keller SM. Intraoperative staging and surgical management of stage IIIA-N2 non-small cell lung cancer. Thorac Surg Clin 2008;18:381–91.

41. Leo F, De Pas T, Catalano G, et al. Re: Randomized controlled trial of resection versus radiotherapy after induction chemotherapy in stage IIIA-N2 non small-cell lung cancer. J Natl Cancer Inst 2007;99:1210–1.

42. Venuta F, Anile M, Diso D, et al. Operative complications and early mortality after induction therapy for lung cancer. Eur J Cardiothorac Surg 2007;31:714–7.

43. Evans NR 3rd, Li S, Wright CD, et al. The impact of induction therapy on morbidity and operative mortality after resection of primary lung cancer. J Thorac Cardiovasc Surg 2010;139:991–6. e1–2.

44. van Meerbeeck JP, Kramer GW, Van Schil PE, et al, European Organisation for Research and Treatment of Cancer-Lung Cancer Group. Randomized controlled trial of resection versus radiotherapy after induction chemotherapy in stage IIIA-N2 non-small-cell lung cancer. J Natl Cancer Inst 2007;99:442–50.

45. Albain KS, Swann RS, Rusch VW, et al. Radiotherapy plus chemotherapy with or without surgical resection for stage III non-small cell lung cancer: a phase III randomized trial. Lancet 2009;374:379–86.

46. Tieu BH, Sanborn RE, Thomas CR. Neoadjuvant therapy for resectable non-small cell lung cancer with mediastinal nodal involvement. Thorac Surg Clin 2008;18:403–15.

47. Burdett SS, Stewart LA, Rydzewska L. Chemotherapy and surgery versus surgery alone in non-small cell lung cancer. Cochrane Database Syst Rev 2007;3:CD006157.

48. Depierre A, Milleron B, Moro-Sibilot D, et al. Preoperative chemotherapy followed by surgery compared with primary surgery in resectable stage I (except T1N0), II, and IIIa non-small-cell lung cancer. J Clin Oncol 2002;20:247–53.

49. Beghmans T, Paesmans M, Meert AP, et al. Survival improvement in resectable non-small-cell lung cancer with (neo)adjuvant chemotherapy: results of a meta-analysis of the literature. Lung Cancer 2005;49:13–23.

50. Burdett S, Stewart LA, Rydzewska L. A systematic review and meta-analysis of the literature: chemotherapy and surgery versus surgery alone in non-small cell lung cancer. J Thorac Oncol 2006;1: 611–21.

51. Gilligan D, Nicolson M, Smith I, et al. Preoperative chemotherapy in patients with resectable non-small cell lung cancer: results of the MRC LU22/NVALT 2/EORTC 08012 multicentre randomised trial and update of systematic review. Lancet 2007; 369(9577):1929–37.

52. Kunitoh H, Kato H, Tsuboi M, et al, Japan Clinical Oncology Group. Phase II trial of preoperative chemoradiotherapy followed by surgical resection in patients with superior sulcus non-small-cell lung cancers: report of Japan Clinical Oncology Group trial 9806. J Clin Oncol 2008;26:644–9.

53. American College of Radiology. ACR appropriateness criteria. Induction and adjuvant therapy for N2 non-small cell lung cancer. 2010. Available at: http://www.acr.org/SecondaryMainMenuCategories/quality_safety/app_criteria/pdf/ExpertPanelonRadiationOncologyLungWorkGroup/InductionandAdjuvantTherapyforN2NonSmallCellLungCancerDoc2.aspx. Accessed September 7, 2011.

54. Cerfolio RJ, Bryant AS. Restaging after neoadjuvant chemoradiotherapy for N2 non-small cell lung cancer. Thorac Surg Clin 2008;18:417–21.

Chest Wall Sarcomas and Induction Therapy

John C. Kucharczuk, MD

KEYWORDS

• Chest wall • Sarcoma • Induction therapy • Tumor

Chest wall sarcomas are uncommon in clinical practice. However, only a small number of surgeons have a working knowledge of the cause, evaluation, treatment, and prognosis of patients with primary or secondary chest wall sarcomas. Often, this unfamiliarity leads to inappropriate diagnostic studies, delays in treatment, and frustration for the patient and surgeon alike. In most instances, early referral to a specialized center with experience in these unusual chest wall tumors should be considered. In addition, although there are extensive formal guidelines for treatment, including the use of multimodality treatment of extremity and retroperitoneal sarcomas, because of the rarity of chest wall sarcomas, no such formal guidance is available.

This article reviews the clinical presentation, diagnostic procedures required for evaluation, and the overall treatment strategy for patients presenting with chest wall sarcomas. The limited situations in which induction therapy before resection is appropriate are discussed. This article provides an approach to streamlining the evaluation and treatment of patients with chest wall sarcoma.

PATHOLOGY

Sarcomas are malignancies arising in connective and supportive tissues. The chest wall contains several distinct tissues at risk for sarcoma development, including fat, muscle, bone, cartilage, and blood vessels. The chest wall is also in close proximity to several organs that may seem to be a palpable chest wall sarcoma by direct extension. These organs include extension from the breast, the lung, and the mediastinum. In addition, because of the large surface area of the chest wall, it can be the site of metastasis from a distant sarcoma; however, pulmonary parenchyma metastasis remains the most common site. The primary framework for classification of chest wall sarcoma is shown in **Box 1**.

CLINICAL EVALUATION

The initial evaluation of these patients begins with a careful history, noting the symptoms associated with the mass and the history of its growth. Prior radiographs, if available, are reviewed to determine the rapidity of the growth. On physical examination, it is important to rule out other sites of distant disease as well as to delineate the proximity to vital structures and to determine the patient's fitness to undergo aggressive therapy. The most common study on presentation is a chest radiograph and a computed tomography (CT) scan of the chest. For those lesions in proximity to vital structures such as the brachial plexus, magnetic resonance imaging is useful to delineate tissue planes and surgical relationships.[1] No radiographic test can delineate a benign and malignant chest wall mass, and a definite diagnosis of chest wall sarcoma cannot be made on any imaging study.

An important management decision is whether or not a preoperative tissue diagnosis is required. This decision is particularly important in those, albeit limited, situations in which induction treatment should be considered.

For small chest wall lesions less than 3 cm, an excisional biopsy with wide margins is often performed for diagnosis and will likely be acceptable for treatment purposes. When a lesion is 3 cm or larger, resection carries a higher morbidity. Additional considerations include the potential need for extensive reconstruction and resultant functionality. In some cases, there may be a role for induction therapy. In this situation, it is advisable to obtain a preoperative tissue diagnosis. Possible

Division of Thoracic Surgery, Hospital of the University of Pennsylvania, 3400 Spruce Street, Philadelphia, PA 19104, USA
E-mail address: john.kucharczuk@uphs.upenn.edu

Thorac Surg Clin 22 (2012) 77–81
doi:10.1016/j.thorsurg.2011.08.015
1547-4127/12/$ – see front matter © 2012 Published by Elsevier Inc.

Box 1
Framework for classification of primary and secondary chest wall sarcomas

Primary sarcoma of the chest wall

Soft tissue sarcoma

Bone and cartilage sarcoma

Secondary masses of the chest wall

Tumor invasion from contiguous breast, lung, or mediastinum

Metastasis from distant sarcoma sites to the chest wall

Box 2
Primary malignant chest wall masses according to tissue of origin

Chest wall sarcomas: soft tissue

Liposarcoma

Rhabdomyosarcoma

Leiomyosarcoma

Malignant fibrous histiocytoma

Angiosarcoma

Chest wall sarcomas: cartilage and bone

Chondrosarcoma

Osteosarcoma

Ewing sarcoma

Synovial cell sarcoma

---

approaches include percutaneous fine-needle aspiration, core needle biopsy, or incision biopsy.

The usefulness of fine-needle aspiration for tissue diagnosis of any chest wall mass, including chest wall sarcomas, remains debated. On the positive side, a fine-needle aspiration is an outpatient procedure that can be performed on the patient's initial visit with little or no morbidity. Although this approach has been reported as an effective technique in these situations in our routine clinical practice, we often find the cytology of fine-needle aspirate is reported as nondiagnostic.[2,3] An alternative is a core needle biopsy, which provides tissue for histologic evaluation, as does the traditional incisional biopsy, often yielding the definitive diagnosis. In keeping with standard principles of sarcoma surgery, it is important to perform core and incisional procedures in a manor that allows excision of the biopsy track at the time of definitive resection. A tissue diagnosis is required in all cases considering induction therapy.

PRIMARY SOFT TISSUE SARCOMAS

There are diverse types of primary sarcoma of the chest wall as listed in **Box 2**.

PRIMARY SARCOMAS OF THE CHEST WALL: SOFT TISSUE

Primary malignant soft tissue sarcomas of the chest wall are generally reported in small series that also include lesions arising in bone and cartilage. Gordon and colleagues[4] reported the largest surgical series of patients with soft tissue sarcomas of the chest wall in 1991. The study included 149 patients who had undergone resection at the Memorial Sloan-Kettering Cancer Center in New York. The 5-year overall survival rate was 66%. The study also included 32 patients who had desmoid tumors, which are not

histologically classified as sarcomas or as malignant. A large retrospective study containing 55 surgically treated patients with soft tissue sarcomas of the chest wall was reported from a single institution in Brazil in 2005.[5] In this series, fibrosarcoma accounted for nearly 53% of the cases. With wide surgical resection they reported disease-free survival rates of 75% at 5 years and 64% at 10 years. Histologic grade of the tumor and the type of surgical resection were found to be independent prognostic factors for disease-free survival. This finding is in keeping with other studies that suggest that age, gender, symptoms, and size do not significantly affect survival.[6]

Liposarcomas commonly present as retroperitoneal masses or extremity masses; primary liposarcomas of the chest wall are exceedingly rare. Most chest wall liposarcomas are low grade and wide surgical resection with a 4 cm R0 resection is considered the optimal treatment; attempts at debulking are considered palliative and offer little advantage to the patient.[7] The role of preoperative adjuvant radiation on the initial presentation of a chest wall liposarcoma is not defined. Radiation therapy is often reserved for patients with recurrent disease who are then offered radical reoperative surgery requiring complex reconstructions.[8] Likewise, at present, there does not seem to be any role for induction chemotherapy. However, there is an interesting report of complete regression of an anterior chest wall liposarcoma with the administration of interferon-α and tumor necrosis factor-α. However, there has not been any follow-up report or duplication of the results.[9]

Rhabdomyosarcoma tumors arise from a primitive muscle rhabdomyoblast. These tumors are found in pediatric populations. The major sites of presentation include the head and neck, the genitourinary system, and the extremities, and the least likely is the chest wall and lungs. From a surgical perspective, the management of patients with rhabdomyosarcoma of the chest wall follows the general surgical principle of a wide local excision to achieve an R0 resection. If there is not a reasonable expectation of obtaining native margins, the National Cancer Institute treatment recommendations suggest considering chemotherapy with or without radiation therapy. This treatment often renders the lesion resectable with negative margins, thus providing good overall survival.[10,11]

Currently, no good data are available to recommend routine induction therapy for chest wall sarcomas, although this has become commonplace in the management of soft tissue sarcomas of the extremities and large retroperitoneal masses. It seems that the most prudent approach is resection when there is a reasonable expectation of a complete resection, and consideration of some type of induction therapy if an R0 resection seems unlikely.

This was borne out in a single-institutional experience with primary chest wall sarcomas reported from MD Anderson in 2001.[12] This retrospective review included patients with sarcomas of soft tissue, cartilage, and bone, as well as desmoid tumors. Nevertheless, the cumulative 5-year survival was 64%, which is to be expected from surgery alone. In adult patients with locally advanced chest wall sarcoma who are not surgical candidates, it may be reasonable to extrapolate from the guidelines for treatment of patients with inoperable sarcomas in general. These guidelines suggest that "in patients with symptomatic, locally-advanced, or inoperable soft tissue sarcoma, in whom tumor response might potentially result in reduced symptomatology or render a tumor resectable, it is reasonable to use ifosfamide in combination with doxorubicin."[13]

PRIMARY SARCOMAS OF THE CHEST WALL: CARTILAGE AND BONE

Chondrosarcoma is the most common primary malignant tumor of the chest wall. It is found along the anterior sternal border or the costochondral arches and presents with pain. It is more common in men than in women. The primary imaging study is a CT scan, but there are no distinguishing radiographic characteristics to provide a definitive diagnosis.[14] Complete surgical resection with adequate surgical margins and immediate reconstruction is the treatment of choice. The Mayo Clinic experience reported in 2004 found a 100%

5-year survival rate and a recurrence rate of less than 10% in patients with adequate surgical margins.[15] In contrast, patients with inadequate surgical margins had a 50% 5-year survival rate and a 75% local recurrence rate. In general, these tumors are considered resistant to chemotherapy and radiation therapy because of their slow growth rate. Nevertheless, new information describing the genetic mutations that occur during the genesis of these tumors may provide a new test for prognosis and potentially a novel target for molecular intervention. In a recently published paper, insulinlike growth factor binding protein 3, which is a known target of P53, has been found to mediate apoptosis with another gene found in chondrosarcomas. Because the rate of apoptosis is lower in chondrosarcomas, this gene combination may serve as a biomarker for prognosis and, potentially, a target for future molecular therapy.[16]

Ewing sarcoma is an aggressive primary malignant bone tumor that presents in children and adolescents. It is more common in boys than in girls and usually presents between the ages of 10 and 20 years. Ewing sarcoma was initially distinguished from osteosarcoma because of its sensitivity to radiation. Although the origin of Ewing sarcoma is not clear, there seems to be a spectrum of tumors that share the same genetic translocation and are referred to as the Ewing family of tumors.[17] Current molecular genetic studies[18] suggest that these small round cell tumors arise from the same primordial bone marrow–derived mesenchymal stem cell.[19,20] These tumors are best referred to as the Ewing sarcoma family of tumors (ESFT).

The initial role of surgery in primary chest wall ESFT is to obtain tissue for diagnosis. Before any procedure, the patient should undergo a full extent-of-disease work-up to rule out distant metastatic disease. When considering a biopsy, it is important to coordinate with the radiation therapist to ensure that the access site will be included in potential future radiation portals. With smaller rib lesions, this may be in the form of a complete excisional biopsy; however, this scenario is extremely rare because most of these tumors present as a sizable mass. Therapeutically, these tumors are best approached with multimodality treatment including preoperative chemotherapy followed by complete resection of residual disease.[21] A 2003 review of 3 multi-institutional trials from the Pediatric Oncology Group suggests that the likelihood of a complete resection is improved with neoadjuvant chemotherapy followed by delayed resection in patients with Ewing sarcoma and closely related primitive neuroectodermal tumors of the chest wall.[22] The definitive resection is undertaken after

4 cycles of chemotherapy. If the resection is complete and the pathologic margins are negative, no radiation therapy is given. The avoidance of radiation therapy may be particularly important in children and adolescents who are at significant risk (10%–30%) of developing a radiation-induced malignancy.[23] Askin tumors are members of the Ewing family of tumors. They are small round cell tumors of the thoracopulmonary region that are within the ESFT and arise from the same primordial stem cells. They are best managed by diagnostic biopsy and preoperative chemotherapy followed by complete surgical resection.[24]

Synovial sarcomas are uncommon but may arise on the trunk where they present as palpable chest wall mass. Although referred to as synovial cell sarcomas, this is a misnomer and the lesions do not arise from synovial cells or joint cavities. They were originally named based on the appearance under light microscopy; however, these tumors are now known to arise from a primitive mesenchymal cell.[25] The most important prognostic factor is tumor size.[26] Limited data suggest that, although there may be an objective response to neoadjuvant chemotherapy, there is no detectable benefit on survival.[27] The current recommendation is aggressive surgical resection. Those with very large tumors or positive surgical margins receive postoperative adjuvant treatment. A potential future therapy may be adoptive immunotherapy. A recent report showed the effectiveness of using an adoptive immunotherapy strategy to treat patients with metastatic melanoma and metastatic synovial cell sarcoma.[28] In this study, patients received their own genetically engineered cell expressing a T cell receptor that recognized the NY-ESO-1 cancer-testes antigen. The NY-ESO-1 antigen is expressed on 80% of synovial cell sarcomas and represents a novel target for treatment. In the study, 4 of 6 patients (67%), with synovial cell sarcoma had measurable tumor regression. In the future, such strategies may be used as induction therapies before surgery to allow more complete resections or after surgery in an adjuvant setting to decrease recurrence rates.

At present, there are no specific guidelines available to aide in the treatment of patients with synovial cell sarcoma of the chest.

SPECIAL CONSIDERATIONS

Primary sarcoma of the lung invading the chest wall does occur but seems to be an infrequent event. In a series lasting more than 16 years, only 18 patients underwent resection for primary lung sarcoma and, of those patients, 3 required en bloc chest wall resection.[29] The investigators concluded that completeness of resection was the most important factor in survival and they suggested that preoperative chemotherapy may be useful in those cases in which complete resection is unlikely based on initial evaluation.

There are a small number of women who present late following chest wall irradiation for the treatment of breast cancer and later develop a radiation-induced sarcoma. From a technical standpoint, wide local R0 resections with reconstructions, when feasible, likely offer the best chance for control and prolonged survival. In some cases, preoperative adjuvant chemotherapy may be useful, but this is usually decided on a case-by-case basis.[30]

Primary breast sarcomas are extremely rare. In one large review from the Mayo Clinic spanning from 1910 to 2000, only 25 women with primary breast sarcoma were identified.[31] This represented only 0.0006% of breast malignancies treated. It is unclear how often primary sarcomas of the breast invade the chest wall, but, in general, these tumors advance by local invasion rather than nodal metastasis.

SUMMARY

Chest wall sarcomas are unusual in clinical practice. Most surgeons have little experience to evaluate and treat patients with chest wall sarcoma. In general, it is important to move quickly to a tissue diagnosis in the evaluation of these patients because physical examination and radiographic study cannot distinguish the histologic type of the lesion. Management of these tumors requires consultation with a highly specialized pathologist to make the correct diagnosis as well as a medical oncologist and radiation therapist to assist in treatment planning. Because of the rarity of these tumors and the consequent lack of data, there are no specific guidelines to guide therapy. However, for those lesions that are small, and for which the morbidity of surgery and loss of functionality are not an issue, no neoadjuvant therapy should be used. In situations in which the morbidity is prohibitive, loss of functionality an issue, or ability to obtain a negative margin unlikely, neoadjuvant therapy should be considered. In these settings, current guidelines for tumors of similar histology, albeit in different locations, should be considered.

REFERENCES

1. Fortier M, Mayo JR, Swensen SJ, et al. MR imaging of chest wall lesions. Radiographics 1994;14:597–606.

2. Gattuso P, Castelli MJ, Reyes CV, et al. Cutaneous and subcutaneous masses of the chest wall: a fine-needle aspiration study. Diagn Cytopathol 1996;15(5):374–6.

3. Shenoy S, Cassim R. Core needle biopsy for diagnosis of giant thoracic liposarcoma. Am Surg 2010; 76(5):E33–4.

4. Gordon MS, Hadju SI, Bains MS, et al. Soft tissue sarcomas of the chest wall. J Thorac Cardiovasc Surg 1991;101:843–54.

5. Gross JL, Younes RN, Haddad FJ, et al. Soft-tissue sarcomas of the chest wall: prognostic factors. Chest 2005;127:902–8.

6. King RM, Pairolero PC, Trastek VF, et al. Primary chest wall tumors: factors affecting survival. Ann Thorac Surg 1986;41:597–601.

7. Fernandez EL, Plasencia LD, Palma JP, et al. Giant ulcerated pleomorphic liposarcoma of the chest wall. J Thorac Oncol 2007;2(12):1126–7.

8. Rocco G, Fazioli F, Cerra R, et al. Composite reconstruction with cryopreserved fascia lata, single mandibular titanium plate, and polyglactin mesh after redo surgery and radiation therapy for recurrent chest wall liposarcoma. J Thorac Cardiovasc Surg 2011;141(3):839–40.

9. Iwagaki H, Hizuta A, Yoshino T, et al. Complete regression of advanced liposarcoma of the anterior chest wall with interferon-alpha and tumor necrosis factor-alpha. Anticancer Res 1993;13(1):13–5.

10. Chui CH, Billups CA, Pappo AS, et al. Predictors of outcome in children and adolescents with rhabdomyosarcoma of the trunk–the St Jude Children's Research Hospital experience. J Pediatr Surg 2005;40(11):1691–5.

11. Hayes-Jordan A, Stoner JA, Anderson JR, et al. The impact of surgical excision in chest wall rhabdomyosarcoma: a report from the Children's Oncology Group. J Pediatr Surg 2008;43(5):831–6.

12. Walsh GL, Davis BM, Swisher SG, et al. A single-institutional, multidisciplinary approach to primary sarcomas involving the chest wall requiring full-thickness resections. J Thorac Cardiovasc Surg 2001;121:48–68.

13. Verma S, Younus J, Stys-Norman D, et al, Sarcoma Disease Site Group. Ifosfamide-based combination chemotherapy in advanced soft tissue sarcoma: a clinical practice guideline. Toronto: Cancer Care Ontario (CCO); 2006. p. 28. (Evidence-based series; no. 11-4).

14. Murphey MD, Flemming DJ, Boyea SR, et al. Enchondroma versus chondrosarcoma in the appendicular skeleton: differentiating features. Radiographics 1998; 5:1213–37.

15. Fong YC, Pairolero PC, Sim FH, et al. Chondrosarcoma of the chest wall. Clin Orthop Relat Res 2004; 427:184–9.

16. Ho L, Stojanovski A, Whetstone H, et al. Gli2 and p53 cooperate to regulate IGFBP-3-mediated chondrocyte apoptosis in the progression from benign to malignant cartilage tumors. Cancer Cell 2009;16:126–36.

17. Delattre O, Zucman J, Melot T, et al. The Ewing family of tumors—a subgroup of small-round-cell tumors defined by specific chimeric transcripts. N Engl J Med 1994;331:294–9.

18. Dagher R, Pham TA, Sorbara L, et al. Molecular confirmation of Ewing sarcoma. J Pediatr Hematol Oncol 2001;23(4):221–4.

19. Suvà ML, Riggi N, Stehle JC, et al. Identification of cancer stem cells in Ewing's sarcoma. Cancer Res 2009;69(5):1776–81.

20. Tirode F, Laud-Duval K, Prieur A, et al. Mesenchymal stem cell features of Ewing tumors. Cancer Cell 2007;11(5):421–9.

21. Saenz NC, Hass DJ, Meyer P, et al. Pediatric chest wall Ewing's sarcoma. J Pediatr Surg 2000;35(4): 550–5.

22. Shamberger RC, LaQuaglia MP, Gebhardt MC, et al. Ewing sarcoma/primitive neuroectodermal tumor of the chest wall: impact of initial versus delayed resection on tumor margins, survival and use of radiation therapy. Ann Surg 2003;238(4):563–8.

23. Paulussen M, Ahresn S, Lehnert M, et al. Second malignancies after Ewing tumor treatment in 690 patients from a cooperative German/Austrian/Dutch study. Ann Oncol 2001;12:1619–30.

24. Veronesi G, Spaggiari L, De Pas T, et al. Preoperative chemotherapy is essential for conservative surgery of Askin tumors. J Thorac Cardiovasc Surg 2003;125(2):429.

25. Miettinen M, Virtanen I. Synovial sarcoma: a misnomer. Am J Pathol 1984;117:18–25.

26. Deshmukh R, Mankin H, Singer S. Synovial sarcoma: the importance of size and location for survival. Clin Orthop Relat Res 2004;419:155–61.

27. Singer S, Baldini EH, Demetri GD, et al. Synovial sarcoma: prognostic significance of tumor size, margin of resection and mitotic activity for survival. J Clin Oncol 1996;14(4):1201–8.

28. Robbins PF, Morgan RA, Feldman SA, et al. Tumor regression in patients with metastatic synovial cell sarcoma and melanoma using genetically engineered lymphocytes reactive with NY-ESO-1. J Clin Oncol 2010;32:2537.

29. Porte HL, Metois DG, Leroy X, et al. Surgical treatment of primary sarcoma of the lung. Eur J Cardiothorac Surg 2000;18:136–42.

30. Quadros CA, Vasconcelos A, Andrade R, et al. Good outcome after neoadjuvant chemotherapy and extended surgical resection for a large radiation-induced high-grade breast sarcoma. Int Semin Surg Oncol 2006;3:18.

31. Adem C, Reynolds C, Ingle JN, et al. Primary breast sarcoma: clinicopathologic series from the Mayo Clinic and review of the literature. Br J Cancer 2004;91:237–41.

Induction Therapy for Thymic Malignancies

Avedis Meneshian, MD, Stephen C. Yang, MD*

KEYWORDS

- Thymoma • Thymic carcinoma • Induction therapy
- Neoadjuvant therapy

Thymic malignancies (thymoma and thymic carcinoma) are relatively rare tumors of the chest that express a broad range of biological behaviors. Surgery remains the mainstay of therapy, and complete surgical resection is the primary predictor of long-term survival.[1,2] Although stage-specific overall long-term survival for patients with stage III cancers is significantly lower than that for patients with stage I or II disease, in patients with stage III disease who undergo successful, microscopically margin-negative (R0) surgical resection, survival approaches that of patients with stage I disease[3] (**Table 1**). For early-stage tumors (Masaoka stage I–IIB; **Table 2**), initial therapy with surgical resection to microscopically negative margins is feasible and is the recommended definitive therapeutic modality.[4–8] However, for patients with more advanced disease (stage III or greater), complete surgical extirpation (including contiguous resection of lungs, pericardium, and/or great vessels) with negative margins is more challenging. Whereas most patients with early-stage disease can undergo R0 resection, only 50% to 60% of patients with stage III thymomas taken directly to surgery can successfully be resected to microscopically negative margins.[9–12] It is in the latter subset of patients that induction therapy plays a role.

Although paradigms for adjuvant chemotherapy and radiation for advanced-stage thymomas and thymic carcinomas are well described,[13] the specific role of neoadjuvant therapy for these malignancies is unclear. The rarity of these tumors and the role of surgery as the traditional mainstay of therapy have resulted in a paucity of clinical trials assessing the value of induction therapy for these cancers. There are no randomized controlled clinical trials aimed to assess the benefit of induction therapy, either directly comparing rates of R0 resection with or without induction therapy, or assessing the long-term survival benefits, and we have to extrapolate from the literature to generate Category 2A recommendations for treatment. Nevertheless, reasonable conclusions can be gleaned by careful examination of the existing literature.

SHOULD PATIENTS WITH STAGE III OR GREATER THYMIC MALIGNANCIES RECEIVE INDUCTION CHEMOTHERAPY OR RADIATION?

To answer this question on the basis of the existing literature, several important end points must be examined. Because an R0 resection is the single most important factor for long-term success in the treatment of thymic malignancies, the immediate question is whether or not induction therapy increases the chances for R0 resection. This is difficult to glean when reviewing large numbers of nonrandomized trials. In such an assessment, the selection criteria used to proceed to surgical resection in patients with stage III or greater disease are a significant confounding variable. The rates of R0 resection in patients undergoing attempted curative resection seem higher if patients are carefully selected for surgery, as in the case of studies aimed at assessing the value of induction chemotherapy or chemoradiation, as compared with retrospective analyses of surgical

Division of Thoracic Surgery, The Johns Hopkins Medical Institutions, 600 North Wolfe Street, Blalock 240, Baltimore, MD 21287, USA
* Corresponding author.
E-mail address: syang7@jhmi.edu

Thorac Surg Clin 22 (2012) 83–89
doi:10.1016/j.thorsurg.2011.09.008
1547-4127/12/$ – see front matter © 2012 Published by Elsevier Inc.

Table 1
Stage-specific overall 10-year survival and survival after complete (R0) surgical resection

Stage	Overall 10-Year Survival (%)	10-Year Survival After R0 Resection (%)
I	80	80
II	78	78
III	47	75
IVA	30	42

Data from Regnard J-F, Magdeleinat P, Dromer C, et al. Prognostic factors and long-term results after thymoma resection: a series of 307 patients. J Thorac Cardiovasc Surg 1996;112:376–84.

outcomes alone serving as historical controls. Such selection bias variability between studies may be standardized in part by assessing what percentage of patients who receive induction therapy in a given study actually make it to surgery, but this information is not clearly defined in any given study. Another important and immediate end point is the degree of clinical/radiographic response to therapy (complete response, partial response, stable disease, or disease progression). If consistent clinically apparent responses can be obtained with induction therapy, one might assume that this would translate into higher rates of R0 resection and consequently greater overall survival. As for patients who have stable disease through induction therapy, even the more aggressive thymic malignancies are generally more indolent than lung or esophageal cancers, and differentiating stable disease from disease progression may be difficult because of the short course of many of these studies. Distinguishing the relative value of chemotherapy, radiation therapy, or both in the neoadjuvant setting remains a challenge, and there are no studies that stratify the relative value of these interventions. Despite these inherent shortcomings, a brief review of the existing literature might help us to ascertain the value of induction therapy for patients with stage III or greater thymic malignancy.

Table 3 summarizes several existing induction therapy trials and provides a synopsis of the relative value of induction therapy (chemotherapy, radiation therapy, or chemoradiation) based on the clinical/radiographic response rates, rates of R0 resection, and overall survival. This discussion relates only to advanced-stage (III–IVB) thymic malignancies, because the current recommendation for stage I to IIB lesions is to proceed directly to surgical resection.[13] This discussion also treats advanced-stage thymomas and thymic carcinomas as a single entity; although this has inherent shortcomings, the WHO classification[14] suggests that this is a continuum of the same disease, and there is sufficient overlap in the advanced stages of these entities by way of outcomes and available therapies that supports this discussion. A summary of most of the relevant studies is shown in **Table 3**. A study by Bretti and colleagues[15] is discussed in greater detail to highlight the relative value of the conclusions of such studies and their shortcomings.

Bretti and colleagues[15] reported a series of 63 patients with malignant thymoma who were treated

Table 2
Modified Masaoka clinical staging of thymic malignancies

Masaoka Stage	Diagnostic Criteria
I	Macroscopically and microscopically completely encapsulated
II	(A) Microscopic transcapsular invasion (B) Macroscopic invasion into surrounding fatty tissue or grossly adherent to but not through mediastinal pleura or pericardium
III	Macroscopic invasion into neighboring organs (pericardium, great vessels, lungs)
IV	(A) Pleural or pericardial dissemination (B) Lymphogenous or hematogenous metastasis

From Masaoka A, Monden Y, Nakahara K, et al. Follow-up study of thymomas with special reference to their clinical stages. Cancer 1981;48:2485–92; with permission.

with a multimodality regimen, which in some included an induction therapy paradigm. Of the 63 patients included in the study, 43 had Masaoka stage III disease and 20 had stage IVA disease. The thymomas in 33 patients with advanced-stage disease were deemed initially unresectable, and the patients were referred for induction therapy (30 underwent surgical resection as the initial therapy and served as the internal control group). Of the 33 patients who received induction therapy, 8 received radiation therapy alone, and 25 received induction chemotherapy alone (18 received a regimen of doxorubicin, cisplatin, vincristine, and cyclophosphamide, and 7 received cisplatin and etoposide), all for a planned 4 cycles of therapy. No patient received concurrent chemoradiation in the neoadjuvant setting. Of the 25 patients who received induction chemotherapy, 2 (8%) had a complete clinical/radiographic response, 16 (64%) had a partial response, 6 (24%) had radiographically stable disease, and 1 (4%) had disease progression. Fourteen of the 25 patients who had induction chemotherapy were then taken to surgery (56% were deemed eligible for resection on secondary surgical evaluation), and 11 of these 14 (76%) patients successfully achieved complete R0 surgical resection. These results represented a 76% R0 resection rate in patients selected for surgical resection after induction chemotherapy, compared with a 67% (20 of 30) R0 resection rate in patients who underwent immediate surgical resection. Of the 8 patients who received induction radiation therapy alone (24–30 Gy), 3 were subsequently considered candidates for resection and 1 (33%) had a successful R0 surgical resection. All patients subsequently received radiation therapy in the adjuvant setting, up to 45 Gy if they had had a complete R0 resection and up to 50 to 60 Gy if they were not surgical candidates or had undergone resection without clear margins. Overall 5-year survival was in the range of 65% to 70% for patients who had margin-negative resection, either directly with surgery or after an induction therapy paradigm; and only 25% if a margin-negative resection could not be achieved. This study confirms that margin-negative resection affords optimal long-term survival even with advanced-stage disease, that immediate surgical resection is reasonable in patients with advanced-stage disease provided an R0 resection can be achieved at the time of resection, and that in patients in whom R0 resection cannot be achieved as the initial therapy, induction paradigms of chemotherapy and/or radiation can potentially increase the chance of subsequent R0 resections (in carefully selected patients) and improve overall survival.

DISCUSSION

Despite a paucity of clinical trials that directly address the role of induction chemotherapy and/or radiation therapy in the treatment of thymic malignancies, the preponderance of existing data suggests that for advanced-stage disease, induction therapy should be strongly considered. The theoretical advantages of therapy in the neoadjuvant setting include improved tolerance of chemotherapy and radiation, potential sterilization of tumor (even with partial responses) with a theoretical reduction of tumor spillage and consequent local recurrence, a more rapid initiation of systemic therapy for the treatment of occult metastatic disease, and the ability to assess therapeutic responsiveness to systemic therapy to guide ongoing therapy decisions in the adjuvant setting. In addition, the existing data suggest that the rates of R0 resection may be greater (60%–80%; see **Table 3**) than the traditionally reported rates[9–12] (50%–60%) after immediate surgical resection for stage III disease. Clinically appreciable response rates (partial clinical/pathologic and complete clinical/radiographic responses) range from 60% to 100% (see **Table 3**), which may translate into higher degrees of R0 resection after induction therapy. Moreover, long-term survival seems more favorable, compared with the overall survival reported in patients with stage III and IV disease.

Nevertheless, there are no sufficient definitive data to support the notion that every patient with stage III or greater disease should first receive induction chemotherapy or radiation, and it remains imperative that every patient with such a thymic malignancy undergo careful assessment by a group of surgeons and medical and radiation oncologists who have expertise in treating patients with thymic malignancies. There will be a handful of patients, who despite having unequivocal stage III disease on workup, might have a very high R0 resection rate with immediate surgery. Local involvement of a portion of the right upper lobe, for example, might represent a carefully selected patient in whom immediate resection with microscopically negative margins might be a very practical first step. The key factors to remember are that an R0 resection is imperative, and therefore careful selection of patients with advanced-stage disease who can undergo immediate surgery must be made by a team of physicians with experience in treating thymic malignancies. The remainder of patients with advanced-stage disease should be considered in an induction therapy paradigm.

Table 3
Summary of various clinical studies on the role of induction therapy for thymic malignancies

Reference	Stage	Induction Chemotherapy	Induction Radiation Therapy	N (No. of Patients with Induction Rx)	Response Rate	R0 Resection Rate	Survival
Yokoi et al[16,17]	III–IVB	CAMP	No	17	CR, 1 (6%) PR, 13 (76%) SD, 3 (18%) DP, none	NR	81% (5 y)
Wright et al[18]	III–IVA	EP	40–45 Gy	10	CR, none PR, 4 (40%) SD, 6 (60%) DP, none	8/10 (80%) (All 10 resected)	69% (5 y)
Lucchi et al[19]	III–IVA	EP + epirubicin	No	30	CR, 2 (7%) PR, 20 (67%) SD, 8 (27%) DP, none	23/30 (77%) (All 30 resected)	86% (10 y, III) 76% (10 y, IVA)
Macchiarini et al[20]	IIIA	EP + epirubicin	No	7	CR, none PR, 7 (100%) SD, none DP, none	4/7 (57%) (All 7 resected)	80% (2 y)
Jacot et al[21]	III, IV	CAP	No	8	CR, none PR, 6 (75%) SD, 1 (12.5%) DP, 1 (12.5%)	2/3 (67%) (3 of 8 resected)	NR

Study	Stage	Regimen		N	Response	Resection	Survival
Kim et al[22]	III, IVA–IVB	CAP + prednisone	No	22	CR, 3 (13.6%) PR, 14 (63.6%) SD, 4 (18%) DP, none	16/21 (76%) (21 of 22 resected)	95% (5 y)
Shin et al[23]	III, IVA	CAP + prednisone	No	12	CR, 3 (25%) PR, 8 (67%) SD, 1 (8%) DP, none	9/11 (81.8%) (11 of 12 resected)	100% (7 y)
Kunitoh et al[24]	III	CODE	No	21	CR, none PR, 13 (62%) SD, 7 (33.3%) DP, 1 (4.8%)	9/13 (69.2%) (13 of 21 resected)	85% (5 y)
Rea et al[25]	III, IVA	ADOC	No	16	CR, 7 (43.8%) PR, 9 (56.3%) SD, none DP, none	11/16 (69%) (16 of 16 resected)	70% (3 y)
Berruti et al[26]	III, IVA	ADOC	No	16	CR, 1 (6.3%) PR, 12 (75%) SD, 2 (12.5%) DP, 1 (6.3%)	9/16 (56%) (16 of 16 resected)	47.5 mo (median)

Abbreviations: ADOC, doxorubicin, cisplatin, vincristine, cyclophosphamide; CAMP, cisplatin, doxorubicin, methylprednisolone; CAP, cisplatin, doxorubicin, cyclophosphamide; CODE, cisplatin, vincristine, doxorubicin, etoposide; CR, complete clinical/radiographic response; DP, disease progression; EP, cisplatin, etoposide; NR, not reported; PR, partial clinical/pathologic response; SD, stable disease.

SUMMARY

A reasonable approach may be as follows, based on an amendment to the National Comprehensive Cancer Network guidelines for thymic malignancies, version 2.2011.[13] Patients with stage I to IIB disease undergo immediate surgical resection, with adjuvant radiotherapy reserved for pathologic capsular invasion or microscopically positive margins (R1 resection). If the final pathology reveals a thymic carcinoma, adjuvant chemotherapy should also be included. Patients who present with stage III to IVA disease proceed to surgery if deemed eligible for resection by a multidisciplinary team of experts in the field of thoracic oncology. However, if it seems unlikely that an R0 resection can be achieved initially, an induction chemotherapy or chemoradiation paradigm should be followed, with restaging after induction therapy and consideration of surgical resectability. If eligible for resection, the patient proceeds to surgery and adjuvant therapy can be considered as described for the early-stage patients; if the thymoma is unresectable, definite chemoradiation is performed.

REFERENCES

1. Maggi G, Casadio C, Cavallo A, et al. Thymoma: results of 241 operated cases. Ann Thorac Surg 1991;51:152–6.
2. Blumberg D, Port JL, Weksler B, et al. Thymoma: a multivariate analysis of factors predicting survival. Ann Thorac Surg 1995;60:908–14.
3. Regnard J-F, Magdeleinat P, Dromer C, et al. Prognostic factors and long-term results after thymoma resection: a series of 307 patients. J Thorac Cardiovasc Surg 1996;112:376–84.
4. Masaoka A. Staging system of thymoma. J Thorac Oncol 2010;5:S304–12.
5. Kondo K, Monden Y. Therapy for thymic epithelial tumors: a clinical study of 1320 patients from Japan. Ann Thorac Surg 2003;76:878–84.
6. Detterbeck FC, Parsons AM. Management of stage I and II thymoma. Thorac Surg Clin 2011;21:59–67.
7. Kondo K. Optimal therapy for thymoma. J Med Invest 2008;55:17–28.
8. Detterbeck FC, Parsons AM. Thymic tumors. Ann Thorac Surg 2004;77:1860–9.
9. Curran WJ Jr, Kornstein MJ, Brooks JJ, et al. Invasive thymoma: the role of mediastinal irradiation following complete or incomplete surgical resection. J Clin Oncol 1988;6(11):1722–7.
10. Ohara K, Okumura T, Sugahara S, et al. The role of preoperative radiotherapy for invasive thymoma. Acta Oncol 1990;29(4):425–9.
11. Akaogi E, Ohara K, Mitsui K, et al. Preoperative radiotherapy and surgery for advanced thymoma with invasion to the great vessels. J Surg Oncol 1996;63(1):17–22.
12. Okumura M, Miyoshi S, Takeuchi Y, et al. Results of surgical treatment of thymomas with special reference to involved organs. J Thorac Cardiovasc Surg 1999;117(3):605–13.
13. National Comprehensive Cancer Network (NCCN). Clinical Practice Guidelines in Oncology. Thymomas and Thymic Carcinomas Version 2. 2011. Available at: http://www.nccn.org/professionals/physician_gls/pdf/thymic.pdf. Accessed November 11, 2011.
14. Kondo K, Yoshizawa K, Tsuyuguchi M, et al. WHO histologic classification is a prognostic factor in thymoma. Ann Thorac Surg 2004;77:1183–8.
15. Bretti S, Berruti A, Loddo C, et al. Multimodal management of stages III–IVa malignant thymoma. Lung Cancer 2004;44(1):69–77.
16. Yokoi K, Matsuguma H, Nakahara R, et al. Multidisciplinary treatment for advanced invasive thymoma with cisplatin, doxorubicin, and methylprednisolone. J Thorac Oncol 2007;2(1):73–8.
17. Ishikawa Y, Mastuguma H, Nakahara R, et al. Multimodality therapy for patients with invasive thymoma disseminated into the pleural cavity: the potential role of extrapleural pneumonectomy. Ann Thorac Surg 2009;88(3):952–7.
18. Wright CD, Choi NC, Wain JC, et al. Induction chemoradiotherapy followed by resection for locally advanced Masaoka stage III and IVA thymic tumors. Ann Thorac Surg 2008;85(2):385–9.
19. Lucchi M, Melfi F, Dini P, et al. Neoadjuvant chemotherapy for stage III and IVA thymomas: a single-institution experience with long follow-up. J Thorac Oncol 2006;1(4):308–13.
20. Macchiarini P, Chella A, Ducci F, et al. Neoadjuvant chemotherapy, surgery, and postoperative radiation therapy for invasive thymoma. Cancer 1991;68(4):706–13.
21. Jacot W, Quantin X, Valette S, et al. Multimodality treatment program in invasive thymic epithelial tumor. Am J Clin Oncol 2005;28(1):5–7.
22. Kim ES, Putnam JB, Komaki R, et al. Phase II study of a multidisciplinary approach with induction chemotherapy, followed by surgical resection, radiation therapy, and consolidation chemotherapy for unresectable malignant thymomas: final report. Lung Cancer 2004;44(3):369–79.
23. Shin DM, Walsh GL, Komaki R, et al. A multidisciplinary approach to therapy for unresectable malignant thymoma. Ann Intern Med 1998;129(2):100–4.
24. Kunitoh H, Tamura T, Shibata T, et al. A phase II trial of dose-dense chemotherapy, followed by surgical resection and/or thoracic radiotherapy, in locally advanced thymoma: report of a Japan Clinical

Oncology Group trial (JCOG 9606). Br J Cancer 2010;103(1):6–11.

25. Rea F, Sartori F, Loy M, et al. Chemotherapy and operation for invasive thymoma. J Thorac Cardiovasc Surg 1993;106(3):543–9.

26. Berruti A, Borasio P, Gerbino A, et al. Primary chemotherapy with adriamycin, cisplatin, vincristine and cylcophosphamide in locally advanced thymomas: a single institution experience. Br J Cancer 1999;81(5):841–5.

Pulmonary Metastasectomy

Francis C. Nichols, MD

KEYWORDS

- Lung metastasis • Pulmonary metastasis
- Pulmonary metastasectomy • Metastasectomy

The inability to prevent and eliminate metastatic disease is a principal reason for cancer death. The presence of metastases often portends uncontrollable tumor spread and subsequent death. The lung is a frequent site of metastatic disease with almost 30% of all patients with cancer eventually developing lung metastases.[1] Nevertheless, the development of one or more new pulmonary nodules in a patient with a prior cancer history does not always portend metastatic disease. A new pulmonary nodule may be benign or represent primary lung cancer in addition to metastatic disease. The likelihood of a new pulmonary nodule being a metastasis or second primary is directly related to the histopathology of the patient's original tumor.[2] For example, if a patient's initial tumor was a sarcoma or melanoma, the new lung nodule is 10 times more likely to be a metastasis than a second primary. If the primary tumor was either colonic or genitourinary in origin, there is a 50% chance that the new nodule is a metastasis. If the primary tumor arose in the head or neck region, then the new lung nodule is only 2 times as likely to be a primary lung cancer as opposed to metastatic.

The initial treatment of metastatic disease often entails chemotherapy; however, surgical pulmonary metastasectomy, for many years, has been advocated in select patients with pulmonary metastasis(es) originating from a variety of solid tumors. Since the first resection of a lung metastasis was reported in 1882,[3] hundreds of articles focusing on pulmonary metastasectomy have been published resulting in the commonly accepted belief that overall survival can be improved by surgical resection of pulmonary metastases.[4–7] This widespread acceptance of the benefits of pulmonary metastasectomy exists despite the fact that most related publications are retrospective reviews involving limited case series with their inherent biases. A widely referenced work is the largest of these reviews: The International Registry of Lung Metastases.[4] This registry gathered data from 5206 patients treated with pulmonary metastasectomy from 18 thoracic surgical units throughout Canada, the United States, and Europe. Survival after complete surgical metastasectomy at 5, 10, and 15 years was 36%, 26%, and 22% respectively. This contrasts with the 5-year and 10-year survival after incomplete pulmonary metastasectomy of 13% and 7%.

Careful analyses of numerous retrospective series have resulted in the general acceptance of selection criteria for patients being considered for surgical pulmonary metastasectomy: definitive control of the primary tumor or the ability to definitively control the primary tumor contemporaneously with control of the pulmonary metastasis(es), the presence of metastasis(es) limited to the lung or elsewhere amenable to complete resection, the ability of the patient to tolerate the planned surgical resection(s), and lack of a better treatment alternative.[8] Prognostic factors warranting consideration before embarking on pulmonary metastasectomy may include the histopathology of the primary tumor, the disease-free interval from initial primary tumor treatment to metastasis development, the presence of other extrathoracic metastases, the number of lung metastases, the tumor doubling time, the presence of lymph node metastases, and, in some cases, the presence of increased levels of serum markers.[8]

thoracic.theclinics.com

Division of General Thoracic Surgery, Mayo Clinic, 200 First Street Southwest, Rochester, MN 55905, USA
E-mail address: nichols.francis@mayo.edu

Thorac Surg Clin 22 (2012) 91–99
doi:10.1016/j.thorsurg.2011.08.017
1547-4127/12/$ – see front matter © 2012 Elsevier Inc. All rights reserved.

Nonetheless, survival after resection of pulmonary metastases remains far from satisfactory and deficiencies clearly exist in our ability to determine which patients might benefit most from surgical pulmonary metastasectomy. The indications for pulmonary metastasectomy continue to evolve and many controversies remain. Recently, the European Society of Thoracic Surgeons (ESTS) conducted the Lung Metastasectomy Project. An international working group was created to address several issues related to pulmonary metastasectomy. Part of this project included a survey of ESTS members regarding pulmonary metastasectomy, which revealed not only areas of practice consistency but also areas of wide variability in daily practice. The ESTS Lung Metastasectomy Project's overarching conclusion was that the level of evidence supporting current practice is too low to set firm recommendations with regard to pulmonary metastasectomy. However, their work was comprehensive enough that a compendium of the ESTS working groups' individual reports was recently published as a series of specially commissioned articles in a supplement of the *Journal of Thoracic Oncology*. These articles form part of the basis for this current review.[9–15] Among the issues addressed are the optimal preoperative imaging studies, the role of mediastinal lymph node staging or dissection, considerations with regard to the surgical approach (eg, video-assisted thoracic surgery [VATS] vs a more traditional open approach), the extent of surgical resection that is acceptable (eg, wedge vs lobectomy vs pneumonectomy), and how pulmonary metastasectomy should be integrated with other treatments. In addition, some of the common tumors prone to metastasizing to the lung are reviewed, and prognostic factors affecting survival and the role of pulmonary metastasectomy in the treatment of these tumors are discussed.

RADIOGRAPHIC IMAGING

Pulmonary metastases have a nonspecific radiographic appearance; nevertheless, imaging is of critical importance for metastasectomy patient selection and for surgical resection planning. Chest computed tomography (CT) is the standard imaging modality for the evaluation of pulmonary nodules. Detterbeck's ESTS workgroup, as part of the Lung Metastasectomy Project, performed a thorough systematic literature review, which led to reasonable guidance with regard to the imaging requirements appropriate for the practice of pulmonary metastasectomy.[11] Among their useful conclusions were:

1. Although 64-, 128-, and 256-slice CT scanners have made chest CT using contiguous volumetric (<0.5 mm) thin sections possible and technologically enticing, currently there are no data supporting the benefit of multidetector CT and volumetric thin section scanning for the radiographic evaluation of patients being considered for pulmonary metastasectomy. However, they do believe that, at a minimum, a helical chest CT scan with a 3-mm to 5-mm slice thickness is recommended.

2. In general, a CT scan should be performed within 4 weeks of pulmonary metastasectomy.

3. If positron emission tomography (PET) is available, it is recommended for patients being considered for pulmonary metastasectomy, especially in situations where the primary tumor would typically be PET avid. The purpose of the PET scan is to rule out occult distant metastases. PET scans in the face of pulmonary metastases are not recommended for the detection of additional pulmonary metastases.

4. Although data are limited, once a pulmonary metastasis(es) is discovered, there does not seem to be a benefit in delaying the time to pulmonary metastasectomy as long as the patient's evaluation is complete. Although some think otherwise, it is clear that pulmonary metastases can further metastasize; 15% to 20% of pulmonary metastasectomy patients are found to have hilar or mediastinal lymph node involvement.[16,17]

5. Because the goal of pulmonary metastasectomy is complete resection of all detectable disease, palpation of the lung(s) is recommended to detect additional metastases beyond those identified on a helical CT scan. Numerous studies have shown that helical CT fails to detect approximately 25% of pulmonary metastases. The working group thought that a thoracoscopic (VATS) approach without palpation was suboptimal unless used as part of a protocol that clearly specified the interval for ongoing CT surveillance and repeat resection, if necessary.

6. There are no controlled studies defining the optimal imaging interval after pulmonary metastasectomy. The workgroup proposed a follow-up baseline scan 4 to 6 weeks after complete metastasectomy if the surgical resection included lung palpation. Additional CT scans are recommended every 6 months for 2 years and then yearly for at least 5 years after metastasectomy. If tumor doubling time is short or if lung palpation was not performed, more frequent follow-up scanning should be considered.

LYMPH NODE STATUS

Although mediastinal lymph node dissection or sampling is a widely accepted standard in pulmonary resection for primary lung cancer,[18] its role during pulmonary metastasectomy has only been clarified in recent years. The International Registry of Lung Metastases found only a 5% incidence of lymph node metastases in 5206 patients undergoing pulmonary metastasectomy.[4] However, it must be recognized that lymph nodes were resected or sampled in only 4.6% of these patients.[4] More recent pulmonary metastasectomy series have helped clarify the incidence of lymph node metastases. In a recent Mayo Clinic pulmonary metastasectomy series, 70 patients had complete mediastinal lymphadenectomy, and lymph node metastases were identified in 20 (28.6%) patients.[16] These were further classified as N1 in 9 (13%) patients, N2 in 8 (11%), and both in 3 (4%). Others have reported similar findings, and the ESTS workgroup dedicated to thoracic lymphatic involvement reviewed data from 6 series encompassing the years 1985 to 2005 and found a weighted average of 22% lymph node metastases at the time of pulmonary metastasectomy for both carcinomas and sarcomas.[13] Internullo and colleagues[19] in their ESTS Pulmonary Metastasectomy workgroup conducted a survey (November 2006 to January 2007) of ESTS members as to their current practice. Regarding preoperative and intraoperative lymph node assessment, their survey demonstrated that a systematic assessment of mediastinal lymph nodes before metastasectomy is uncommon; 43.8% of respondents rarely, 24% never, and 28.8% sometimes performed mediastinoscopy as part of the evaluation of a patient undergoing metastasectomy. Only 3.4% of the survey respondents consistently used mediastinoscopy in the evaluation of mediastinal lymph nodes before performing pulmonary metastasectomy. The ESTS survey also revealed that, at the time of pulmonary metastasectomy, 55.5% of respondents sample mediastinal lymph nodes, 13% perform formal lymphadenectomy, and 3.2% perform no lymph node evaluation at all. The safety of mediastinal lymphadenectomy during major pulmonary resections has been demonstrated in the American College of Surgeons Oncology Group's randomized prospective trial (ACOSOG Z0030).[20]

In our series, the presence of lymph node metastases was found to be a prognostic indicator.[16] Three-year survival for patients without lymph node metastases was 69% compared with only 38% for those with metastases (P<.001) (**Fig. 1**). In our series, there was no survival difference when only N1 lymph nodes were metastatically involved compared with N2 lymph nodes. However, only 2 patients with metastatically involved lymph nodes survived beyond 4 years; both had low-grade renal cell carcinoma. Other investigators

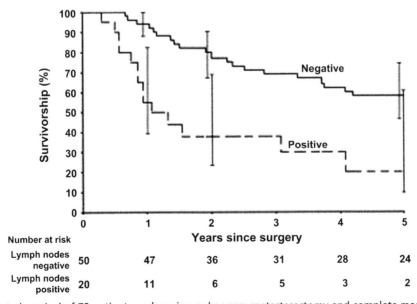

Fig. 1. Estimated survival of 70 patients undergoing pulmonary metastasectomy and complete mediastinal lymphadenectomy without metastatic lymph node involvement (negative) and with lymph node involvement (positive). Zero time on the abscissa is the date of first pulmonary metastasectomy and lymph node dissection (P<.001). (*From* Ercan S, Nichols FC III, Trastek VF, et al. Prognostic significance of lymph node metastasis found during pulmonary metastasectomy for extrapulmonary carcinoma. Ann Thorac Surg 2004;77:1788; with permission.)

have demonstrated a survival difference related to the lymph node stations metastatically involved.[21,22] Pfannschmidt and colleagues,[21] in a series of 245 patients, showed median survival after complete resection was 32.7 months for patients with N1 disease versus 20.6 months for patients with N1 and N2 disease. Welter and colleagues,[22] in 169 patients who had metastasectomy for colorectal cancer, showed statistically significant survival differences of 78.5%, 0%, and 0% for patients with intrapulmonary, hilar, and mediastinal lymph node metastases, respectively. Not all pulmonary metastasectomy series confirm the poor prognosis of metastatic lymph node involvement; however, in most of the series, the extent of lymph node sampling or lymphadenectomy at the time of metastasectomy is difficult to elicit.[23–25]

Although these series were small, where systematic lymph node assessment has been performed as part of pulmonary metastasectomy, it seems clear and is not surprising that patients with demonstrated metastatic lymph node involvement have a much worse survival. However, it is not clear whether there is any survival benefit to lymph node removal, or whether lymphadenectomy merely stages these patients more accurately and, in turn, influences additional oncologic therapy. Before performing pulmonary metastasectomy, appropriate surgical candidates with worrisome

mediastinal lymph nodes should be considered for more formal mediastinal evaluation, which might include endoscopic bronchial ultrasonography (EBUS), esophageal endoscopic ultrasonography (EUS), and mediastinoscopy. However, whether to exclude patients from subsequent pulmonary metastasectomy because of mediastinal lymph node involvement is more controversial, especially with the ever-changing oncologic landscape.[15,19,21,26] What is clearer is that mediastinal lymphadenectomy should be performed in all patients undergoing pulmonary metastasectomy to achieve accurate staging, guide additional treatment, and perhaps improve survival.[27]

CONSIDERATIONS FOR THE SURGICAL APPROACH

Numerous surgical approaches for pulmonary metastasectomy have been described and clearly there are advantages and disadvantages with each. **Table 1** shows the results of the ESTS survey on the respondents' preferred surgical approach. Although sternotomy can provide access to both hemithoraces, visualization, palpation, and resection of lower lobe metastases, particularly the left lower lobe, are problematic and, along with the clamshell approach, are now primarily of historical interest. Molnar and colleagues[12] in their ESTS

Table 1
Results of the ESTS survey regarding the surgical approach for pulmonary metastasectomy

	No. of Patients	(%)
Which is your preferred approach for unilateral metastases		
Anterolateral thoracotomy	53	(36.3)
Video-assisted thoracic surgery (VATS)	42	(28.8)
Posterior muscle sparing thoracotomy	38	(26)
Posterolateral thoracotomy	33	(22.6)
Horizontal axillary thoracotomy	15	(10.3)
Vertical axillary thoracotomy	10	(6.9)
Sternotomy	2	(1.4)
Other	7	(4.8)
Which is your preferred approach for bilateral metastases		
Bilateral staged thoracotomy	96	(66.2)
Sternotomy (1-stage)	39	(26.9)
Bilateral sequential thoracotomy (1-stage)	28	(19.3)
Bilateral staged video-assisted thoracic surgery (VATS)	18	(12.4)
Bilateral video-assisted thoracic surgery (VATS) (1-stage)	11	(7.6)
Clamshell (1-stage)	11	(7.6)
Other	3	(2.1)

Adapted from Intermullo E, Cassivi SD, Van Raemdonck D, et al. Pulmonary metastasectomy a survey of current practice amongst members of the European Society of Thoracic Surgeons. J Thorac Oncol 2008;3:1257–66; with permission.

workgroup considered in depth the surgical approach to pulmonary metastasectomy. They considered 4 clinically relevant questions: (1) Is there evidence that exists for the need for lung palpation? (2) Is there evidence demonstrating a difference in outcome for the open versus VATS approach? (3) Is there evidence of a difference in outcome for initial bilateral exploration versus unilateral exploration? (4) In patients with known bilateral metastases, is there an outcome difference in a simultaneous versus staged approach?

The purported advantages of VATS (excellent visualization of the pleural surfaces, decreased postoperative pain, and decreased length of hospital) stay conflict with the major disadvantage of VATS, that is, the inability to bimanually palpate the entire lung. McCormack and colleagues,[28,29] in 2 separate reviews, found that CT underdetected the true number of metastases. In their later review, they prospectively compared CT, VATS, and confirmatory open thoracotomy with palpation, and a 56% failure rate to detect all metastases was found. Similarly, recent studies by both Ellis and colleagues[30] and Cerfolio and colleagues[31] found that, despite the increased sensitivity of CT imaging, a significant number of pulmonary metastases were found intraoperatively that were not evident on CT and those authors believed that open thoracotomy remains the standard of care for pulmonary metastasectomy. Despite the finding of these additional non-imaged metastases, the clinical significance of this remains uncertain. There are numerous articles demonstrating no difference in survival between the VATS and open approaches.[32–36] Roth and colleagues[37] demonstrated that there was no survival advantage to bilateral lung exploration when imaging revealed only unilateral disease. Similarly, Younes and colleagues[38] found no survival advantage in the performance of bilateral thoracotomies for exploration when unilateral disease is evident. Molnar's workgroup found no randomized controlled or meta-analysis data to support one surgical approach.[12] Nonetheless, the following recommendations were made:

1. Thoracotomy seems to be the preferred approach even with bilateral metastatic disease. For bilateral metastases, sequential thoracotomy with an interval of 3 to 6 weeks is recommended and an interval CT scan is recommended. In our practice, the timing of the sequential thoracotomies depends on the patient's recovery from the initial thoracotomy and performance status. In appropriate patients, the subsequent thoracotomy is often accomplished during the initial hospitalization and thus in a shorter time frame than Molnar's workgroup suggests and without repeat CT.
2. With regard to VATS, the evidence for its superiority is a matter of debate. VATS seems appropriate for diagnostic procedures, but it is not the standard for therapeutic pulmonary metastasectomy. The workgroup concluded that no alternative to palpation currently exists.

EXTENT OF SURGICAL RESECTION

The goal of pulmonary metastasectomy is resection of the metastasis with free margins while simultaneously preserving as much normal lung parenchyma as possible. In the ESTS survey, stapled wedge resection was the most common form of resection (89%), precision excision was the choice of 17.8%, anatomic segmentectomy 4.8%, and lobectomy 2.1%.[19] Two-thirds of survey respondents considered the need for pneumonectomy to be a relative contraindication, and 23% considered pneumonectomy an absolute contraindication to pulmonary metastasectomy. Resection was most commonly performed with surgical staplers (82.2%), electrocautery (32.2%), direct suture (24.7%), and laser (12.3%).

Most reports of pneumonectomy for pulmonary metastasectomy are smaller case series or parts of larger reviews. Within the International Registry of Lung Metastases, 133 patients (2.6%) had pneumonectomy with a perioperative mortality of 4%.[4] In addition, within the registry, Koong and colleagues[39] found that of the 133 primary pneumonectomies, 65 (49%) were performed for epithelial tumors and 43 (33%) for sarcomatous tumors. They found 5-year survival to be 20% if complete resection was performed, and survival was not influenced by histopathology, lymph node status, and the disease-free interval. There seemed to be a survival advantage in patients with a single metastasis. If incomplete resection occurred, the operative mortality was 19% with most not surviving beyond 2 years. In our Mayo Clinic series of completion pneumonectomies performed for a variety of benign and malignant causes, there was no operative mortality and 5-year survival was 41% for the 20 patients undergoing pulmonary metastasectomy.[40] Spaggiari and colleagues[41] reported on 42 patients who underwent pneumonectomy for pulmonary metastasectomy. Operative mortality was 7.1% and morbidity 9.5%. Median survival was 6.5 months ranging between 1 and 144 months, and 5-year survival was 16.8%. Although not an absolute contraindication, the poor long-term outcome for pneumonectomy resulted in the investigators and Pairolero, in his invited commentary, suggesting very strict selection criteria for pneumonectomy for pulmonary metastasectomy: a solitary central lesion in a patient ideally with a previous soft tissue or bone tumor with a long tumor-free interval, who had no previous pulmonary resection for metastatic disease.[41]

Recurrent lung metastases are common. Within the International Registry of Lung Metastases, recurrent disease was found in 53% of all patients undergoing complete resection with the median time to recurrence being 10 months.[4] Sarcomas and melanomas were noted to have a higher rate of recurrence (64%) compared with epithelial or germ cell tumors (46% and 26%, respectively). For patients who had a second metastasectomy, 5-year survival was 44% and 10-year survival was 29%.[4] Five-year survival rates of 33% to 55% have been reported in several series involving recurrent colorectal metastases.[22,26,42] In carefully selected patients, ongoing attempts to regain intrathoracic control of recurrent metastatic disease are supported by many investigators; however, the apparent benefit may be the result of survivor bias. For repeat pulmonary metastasectomy, factors to consider include the histopathology, disease-free interval, and the amount of lung that will need to be resected to accomplish complete metastasectomy.[43]

SOME COMMON PULMONARY METASTASECTOMY TUMOR HISTOPATHOLOGIES
Osteosarcoma

Failure to control intrathoracic disease is the most common cause of death in patients with metastatic osteosarcoma.[44] Nearly 20% of patients with osteogenic sarcoma develop metastatic disease with the lung being the metastatic site in 85% of those patients.[45] Ferrari and colleagues[46] found that favorable prognostic indicators included having 2 or fewer metastases and a disease-free interval longer than 24 months. In 62 patients who had metastatic osteosarcoma at initial presentation, neoadjuvant chemotherapy was followed by pulmonary metastasectomy. Improved survival was found with increasing age, unilateral tumor location, response to neoadjuvant therapy, and the ability to achieve complete resection.[47] Thus, both chemotherapy and surgery play important roles in the treatment of osteosarcoma.[48]

Breast Cancer

In a Mayo Clinic series of 13,502 patients with breast cancer, 60 patients were found with isolated pulmonary metastases.[49] Five-year survival after complete pulmonary metastasectomy was

35.6% compared with 42.1% in patients with incomplete resection. In contrast, in the International Registry of Lung Metastases, 5-year survival after complete pulmonary metastasectomy was 38% versus 16% with incomplete resection.[50] Adjuvant therapies are commonplace in the treatment of breast cancer, making an understanding of the impact of pulmonary metastasectomy difficult. Welter and colleagues[51] suggested that the improvement in survival for patients with pulmonary metastases secondary to metastatic breast cancer is due to chemotherapy and hormonal therapy.

Colorectal Cancer

Extrathoracic metastatic disease is the most common site in colorectal cancer with isolated pulmonary metastases occurring in just 2% of patients.[52] There are no prospective randomized trials for colorectal pulmonary metastasectomy, making evaluation of the effectiveness of this operation challenging. Pfannschmidt and colleagues,[53] in their ESTS workgroup, reported on outcome factors for pulmonary resection in metastatic colorectal cancer. Their systematic review included 15 articles and 1539 patients. Overall 5-year survival after complete surgical resection was 40% to 68%. Five-year disease-free survival ranged from 19.5% to 34.4%. For patients having both hepatic and pulmonary metastasectomy, overall survival was between 31% and 60.8%; estimated disease-free survival at 3 years was 8%.[53] Completeness of resection was the most important prognostic indicator. Kanemitsu and colleagues[54] developed a predictive model for estimating long-term outcome. Primary histopathology, hilar or mediastinal lymph node involvement, number of metastases, preoperative carcinoembryonic antigen level, and the presence of extrathoracic disease were factors used in the calculation of a clinical risk score, which was highly predictive of long-term outcome.

Chemotherapy for the treatment of metastatic colorectal cancer continues to evolve. The impact of neoadjuvant and adjuvant chemotherapy as it relates to pulmonary metastasectomy and long-term survival still has not been sufficiently addressed.[53] In most studies, small patient numbers prevent useful statistical analyses.

Renal Cell Carcinoma

Thirty percent of patients with renal cell cancer present with metastatic disease and between 14% and 29% of patients initially treated for clinically localized disease develop metastatic disease.[55–58] Traditionally, kidney cancers have been resistant to chemotherapy and radiotherapy, and have only shown a limited response to immunotherapy.[59,60] Sunitinib and sorafenib are oral multitargeted tyrosine kinase inhibitors that have recently been trialed for patients with metastatic renal cell carcinoma. An objective response rate of 47% was seen with sunitinib; however, only 3% of patients demonstrated a complete response to therapy and most patients showed partial responses or stabilization of disease.[61] Thus, surgical resection, when technically possible, remains the only potentially curative treatment for metastatic renal cell carcinoma.[60] In a recent Mayo Clinic series, Alt and colleagues[60] demonstrated that for 224 patients with renal cell cancer with only pulmonary metastases, the 5-year cancer-specific survival for patients who had complete metastasectomy was 73.6% compared with 19% for patients who had incomplete resection ($P<.001$).

For patients undergoing pulmonary metastasectomy, completeness of metastasectomy was a significant prognostic indicator in all series, fewer and smaller metastases positively influenced survival, and, in some series, a longer disease-free interval correlated with better survival.[62] The optimal treatment for patients with metastatic renal cell cancer may prove to be the combination of chemotherapy and, in appropriate patients, surgical resection, but further trials are necessary.[60,63–65]

SUMMARY

Patients with untreated metastatic disease have a less than 5% to 10% 5-year survival, and for the patient who has metastatic disease isolated to the lungs, pulmonary metastasectomy remains the best hope for cure.[62] However, despite hundreds of studies over several decades, randomized control data in support of pulmonary metastasectomy are still lacking, and the evidence on which this commonly accepted surgical practice is based is for the most part weak.[66] Under the auspices of the European Society of Thoracic Surgeons, the multinational Lung Metastasectomy Working Group surveyed its membership with regard to their individual metastasectomy practices and conducted systematic literature reviews; the end results being the provision of published guidance with regards to surgical pulmonary metastasectomy.[8–15,19,27,43,53]

REFERENCES

1. Davidson RS, Nwogu CE, Brentjens MJ, et al. The surgical management of pulmonary metastasis: current concepts. Surg Oncol 2001;10:35–42.

2. Rusch VW. Pulmonary metastasectomy: current indications. Chest 1995;107:322S–32S.

3. Weinlechner J. Tumoren an der Brust und deren Behandlung (Resektion der Rippen, Eroeffnung der Brusthoehle, partielle Entfernung der Lunge). Wien Med Wochenschr 1882;20–1 [in German].

4. Pastorino U, Buyse M, Friedel G, et al. Long-term results of lung metastasectomy: prognostic analyses based an 5206 cases. J Thorac Cardiovasc Surg 1997;113:37–49.

5. Martini N, McCormack PM. Evolution of the surgical management of pulmonary metastases. Chest Surg Clin N Am 1998;8:13–27.

6. Allen MS, Putnam JB Jr. Secondary tumors of the lung. In: Shields TW, LoCicero J, Reed CE, et al, editors. General thoracic surgery. 7th edition. Philadelphia: Lippincott Williams & Wilkins; 2009. p. 1619–46.

7. Pastorino U, Grunenwald D. Surgical resection of pulmonary metastases. In: Patterson GA, Cooper JD, Deslauriers J, et al, editors. Pearson's thoracic and esophageal surgery. 3rd edition. Philadelphia: Churchill Livingstone Elsevier; 2008. p. 851–63.

8. Rusch VW. Pulmonary metastasectomy a moving target. J Thorac Oncol 2010;5:S130–1.

9. Van Raemdonck D, Friedel G. The European Society of Thoracic Surgeons lung metastasectomy project. J Thorac Oncol 2010;5:S127–9.

10. Pastorino U, Treasure T. A historical note on pulmonary metastasectomy. J Thorac Oncol 2010;5: S132–3.

11. Detterbeck FC, Grodzki T, Gleeson F, et al. Imaging requirements in the practice of pulmonary metastasectomy. J Thorac Oncol 2010;5:S134–9.

12. Molnar TF, Gebitekin C, Turna A. What are the considerations in the surgical approach in pulmonary metastasectomy? J Thorac Oncol 2010;5: S140–4.

13. Garcia-Yuste M, Cassivi SD, Paleru C. The number of pulmonary metastases: influence on practice and outcome. J Thorac Oncol 2010;5:S161–3.

14. Detterbeck F. The number of metastases and its influence on outcome. Editorial comment. J Thorac Oncol 2010;5:S164–5.

15. Garcia-Yuste M, Cassivi S, Paleru C. Thoracic lymphatic involvement in patients having pulmonary metastasectomy. J Thorac Oncol 2010;5:S166–9.

16. Ercan S, Nichols FC III, Trastek VF, et al. Prognostic significance of lymph node metastasis found during pulmonary metastasectomy for extrapulmonary carcinoma. Ann Thorac Surg 2004;77:1786–91.

17. Loehe F, Kobinger S, Hatz RA, et al. Value of systematic mediastinal lymph node dissection during pulmonary metastasectomy. Ann Thorac Surg 2001;72:225–9.

18. Ponn RB, LoCicero J, Daly BD. Surgical treatment of non-small cell lung cancer. In: Shields TW, LoCicero J, Ponn RB, et al, editors. General thoracic

surgery. 6th edition. Philadelphia: Lippincott Williams & Wilkins; 2005. p. 1548–87.

19. Internullo E, Cassivi SD, Van Raemdonck D, et al. Pulmonary metastasectomy a survey of current practice amongst members of the European Society of Thoracic Surgeons. J Thorac Oncol 2008;3: 1257–66.

20. Allen MS, Darling GE, Pechet TT, et al. Morbidity and mortality of major pulmonary resections in patients with early-stage lung cancer: initial results of the randomized, prospective ACOSOG Z0030 trial. Ann Thorac Surg 2006;81:1013–9.

21. Pfannschmidt J, Klode J, Muley T, et al. Nodal involvement at the time of pulmonary metastasectomy: experience in 245 patients. Ann Thorac Surg 2006;81:448–54.

22. Welter S, Jacobs J, Krbek T, et al. Prognostic impact of lymph node involvement in pulmonary metastases from colorectal cancer. Eur J Cardiothorac Surg 2007;31:167–72.

23. Ike H, Shimada H, Ohiki S, et al. Results of aggressive resection of lung metastases from colorectal carcinoma detected by intensive follow-up. Dis Colon Rectum 2002;45:468–73.

24. Shiono S, Ishii G, Nagai K, et al. Histopathologic prognostic factors in resected colorectal lung metastases. Ann Thorac Surg 2005;79:278–82.

25. Lin BR, Chang TC, Lee YC, et al. Pulmonary resection for colorectal cancer metastases: duration between cancer onset and lung metastasis as an important prognostic factor. Ann Surg Oncol 2009; 16:1026–32.

26. Pfannschmidt J, Muley T, Hoffman H, et al. Prognostic factors and survival after complete resection of pulmonary metastases from colorectal carcinoma: experiences in 167 patients. J Thorac Cardiovasc Surg 2003;126:732–9.

27. Kaifi JT, Gusani NJ, Deshaives I, et al. Indications and approach to surgical resection of lung metastases. J Surg Oncol 2010;102:187–95.

28. McCormack PM, Ginsberg KB, Bains MS, et al. Accuracy of lung imaging in metastases with implications for the role of thoracoscopy. Ann Thorac Surg 1993;56:863–5.

29. McCormack PM, Bains MS, Begg CB, et al. Role of video-assisted thoracic surgery in the treatment of pulmonary metastases: results of a prospective trial. Ann Thorac Surg 1996;62:213–6.

30. Ellis MC, Hessman CJ, Weerasinghe R, et al. Comparison of pulmonary nodule detection rates between preoperative CT imaging and intraoperative lung palpation. Am J Surg 2011;201:619–22.

31. Cerfolio RJ, Bryant AS, McCarty TP, et al. A prospective study to determine the incidence of non-malignant pulmonary nodules in patients who undergo metastasectomy by thoracotomy with lung palpation. Ann Thorac Surg 2011;91:1696–701.

32. Nakas A, Klimatsides MN, Entwisle J, et al. Video-assisted versus open pulmonary metastasectomy: the surgeon's finger or the radiologist's eye? Eur J Cardiothorac Surg 2009;36:469–74.

33. Mutsaerts EL, Zoetmulder FA, Meijer S, et al. Long term survival of thoracoscopic metastasectomy vs. metastasectomy by thoracotomy in patients with a solitary pulmonary lesion. Eur J Surg Oncol 2002;28:864–8.

34. Carballo M, Maish MS, Jaroszewski DE, et al. Video-assisted thoracic surgery (VATS) as a safe alternative for the resection of pulmonary metastases: a retrospective cohort study. J Cardiothorac Surg 2009;4:13.

35. Gossot D, Radu C, Girard P, et al. Resection of pulmonary metastases from sarcoma: can some patients benefit from a less invasive approach? Ann Thorac Surg 2009;87:238–43.

36. Lim MC, Lee HS, Seo SS, et al. Pathologic diagnosis and resection of suspicious thoracic metastases in patients with cervical cancer through thoracotomy or video-assisted thoracic surgery. Gynecol Oncol 2010;116:478–82.

37. Roth JA, Pass HJ, Wesley MN, et al. Comparison of median sternotomy and thoracotomy for resection of pulmonary metastases in patients with adult soft-tissue sarcomas. Ann Thorac Surg 1986;42:134–8.

38. Younes RN, Gross JL, Deheinzelin D. Surgical resection of unilateral lung metastasis: is bilateral thoracotomy necessary? World J Surg 2002;26:1112–6.

39. Koong HN, Pastorino U, Ginsberg RJ. Is there a role for pneumonectomy in pulmonary metastases? Ann Thorac Surg 1999;68:2039–43.

40. McGovern EM, Trastek VF, Pairolero PC, et al. Completion pneumonectomy: indications, complications, and results. Ann Thorac Surg 1988;46:141–6.

41. Spaggiari L, Grunenwald DH, Girard P. Pneumonectomy for lung metastases: indications, risks, and outcomes. Ann Thorac Surg 1998;66:1930–3.

42. Ogata Y, Matono K, Hayashi A. Repeat pulmonary resection for isolated recurrent lung metastases yields results comparable to those after first pulmonary resection in colorectal cancer. World J Surg 2005;29:363–8.

43. Migliore M, Jakovic R, Hensens A, et al. Extending surgery for pulmonary metastasectomy what are the limits? J Thorac Oncol 2010;5:S155–60.

44. Sternberg DI, Sonnet JR. Surgical therapy of lung metastases. Semin Oncol 2007;34:186–96.

45. Kager L, Zoubek A, Potschger U, et al. Primary metastatic osteosarcoma: presentation and outcome of patients treated on neoadjuvant Cooperative Osteosarcoma Study Group protocols. J Clin Oncol 2003; 21:2011–8.

46. Ferrari S, Briccoli A, Mercuri M, et al. Postrelapse survival in osteosarcoma of the extremities: prognostic factors for long-term survival. J Clin Oncol 2003;21:710–5.

47. Meyers PA, Heller G, Healey JH, et al. Osteogenic sarcoma with clinically detectable metastasis at initial presentation. J Clin Oncol 1993;11:449–53.

48. Bacci G, Briccoli A, Longhi A, et al. Treatment and outcome of recurrent osteosarcoma: experience at Rizzoli in 235 patients initially treated with neoadjuvant chemotherapy. Acta Oncol 2005;44:748–50.

49. McDonald ML, Deschamps C, Ilstrup DM, et al. Pulmonary resection for metastatic breast cancer. Ann Thorac Surg 1994;58:1599–602.

50. Friedel G, Pastorino U, Ginsberg RJ, et al. Results of lung metastasectomy from breast cancer: prognostic criteria on the basis of 467 cases of the International Registry of Lung Metastases. Eur J Cardiothorac Surg 2002;22:335–44.

51. Welter S, Jacobs J, Krbek T, et al. Pulmonary metastases of breast cancer. When is resection indicated. Eur J Cardiothorac Surg 2008;34:1228–34.

52. McCormack PM, Burt ME, Bains MS, et al. Lung resection for colorectal metastases. 10-year results. Arch Surg 1992;127:1403–6.

53. Pfannschmidt J, Hoffman H, Dienemann H. Reported outcome factors for pulmonary resection in metastatic colorectal cancer. J Thorac Oncol 2010; 5:S172–8.

54. Kanemitsu Y, Kato T, Hirai T, et al. Preoperative probability model for predicting overall survival after resection of pulmonary metastases from colorectal cancer. Br J Surg 2004;91:112–20.

55. Pantuck AJ, Zisman A, Belldegrun AS. The changing natural history of renal cell carcinoma. J Urol 2001;166:1611–23.

56. Kattan MW, Reuter V, Mortzer RJ, et al. A postoperative prognostic nomogram for renal cell carcinoma. J Urol 2001;166:63–7.

57. Sorbellini M, Kattan MW, Synder ME, et al. A postoperative prognostic nomogram predicting recurrence for patients with conventional clear cell renal cell carcinoma. J Urol 2005;173:48–51.

58. Zisman A, Pantuck AJ, Wieder J, et al. Risk group assessment and clinical outcome algorithm to predict the natural history of patients with surgically resected renal cell carcinoma. J Clin Oncol 2002;20: 4559–66.

59. Motzer RJ, Bacik J, Murphy BA, et al. Interferon-alfa as a comparative treatment for clinical trials of new therapies against advanced renal cell carcinoma. J Clin Oncol 2002;20:289–96.

60. Alt A, Boorjian SA, Lohse CM, et al. Survival after complete surgical resection of multiple metastases from renal cell carcinoma. Cancer 2011;117: 2873–82.

61. Motzer RJ, Hutson TE, Tomczak P, et al. Overall survival and updated M results for sunitinib compared with interferon alfa in patients with metastatic renal cell carcinoma. J Clin Oncol 2009;27: 3584–90.

62. Hornbech K, Ravn J, Steinbrüchel DA. Current status of pulmonary metastasectomy. Eur J Cardiothorac Surg 2011;39:955–62.

63. Cowey CI, Amin C, Pruthi RS, et al. Neoadjuvant clinical trial with sorafenib for patients with stage II or higher renal cell carcinoma. J Clin Oncol 2010; 28:1502–7.

64. Thomas AA, Rini BI, Lane BR, et al. Response of the primary tumor to neoadjuvant sunitinib in patients with advanced renal cell carcinoma. J Urol 2009; 181:518–23.

65. Thomas AA, Rini BI, Stephenson AJ, et al. Surgical resection of renal cell carcinoma after targeted therapy. J Urol 2009;182:881–6.

66. Treasure T. Pulmonary metastasectomy: a common practice based on weak evidence. Ann R Coll Surg Engl 2007;89:744–8.

Management of Barrett Esophagus with High-grade Dysplasia

Thomas W. Rice, MD[a],*, John R. Goldblum, MD[b]

KEYWORDS

- Intestinal metaplasia • Specialized columnar epithelium
- Intramucosal cancer • Mucosal ablation
- Mucosal resection • Esophagectomy

The management of high-grade dysplasia arising in Barrett esophagus is in evolution. Both increasing knowledge of this fascinating disease and new technologies have spurred this process. Many recent guidelines have been published to aid physicians and patients with management decisions.[1–4] An exhaustive guideline presentation is not the purpose of this article. For everyday practice, however, a review of the definitions, diagnosis, surveillance, natural history, management options, and controversies surrounding these areas is critical in managing high-grade dysplasia complicating Barrett esophagus.

DEFINITIONS

The definition of Barrett esophagus varies in different parts of the world. The columnar-lined esophagus can have 3 distinct epithelial types: cardia-type, fundic-type, and intestinal (specialized columnar epithelium).[5] In many countries, the finding of columnar lining in the esophagus, regardless of the type, leads to the diagnosis of Barrett esophagus. The difficulties, however, in defining the esophagogastric junction and distinguishing normal gastric epithelium from metaplastic cardia/fundic-type mucosa in the

esophagus and the long-held belief that only specialized columnar epithelium can progress to cancer[6–8] led physicians in the United States to restrict the diagnosis of Barrett esophagus to the finding of intestinal metaplasia.[9] A recent Irish population-based study confirms that patients with specialized columnar epithelium at index biopsy have the greatest risk of developing esophageal cancer; however, patients with metaplastic cardia-type or fundic-type mucosa without specialized columnar epithelium at index biopsy are also at increased risk.[10] Thus, it is important to confirm which definition of Barrett esophagus is used. Patients with Barrett esophagus containing only metaplastic cardia or fundic-type epithelium should not be ignored.

Dysplasia is defined as neoplastic epithelium confined by the basement membrane of the gland from which it arises. Care must be taken not to equate the term *atypia* with *dysplasia*, because cytologic atypia may be reparative or dysplastic/neoplastic in nature. In the 5-tier system for grading dysplasia in Barrett esophagus (no dysplasia, indefinite for dysplasia, low-grade dysplasia, high-grade dysplasia, and intramucosal cancer), high-grade dysplasia is the most advanced form of intraepithelial neoplasia.

The authors have nothing to disclose.
[a] Department of Thoracic and Cardiovascular Surgery, Cleveland Clinic, 9500 Euclid Avenue/Desk J4-1, Cleveland, OH 44195, USA
[b] Department of Anatomic Pathology, Cleveland Clinic, 9500 Euclid Avenue/Desk L25, Cleveland, OH 44195, USA
* Corresponding author.
E-mail address: ricet@ccf.org

Thorac Surg Clin 22 (2012) 101–107
doi:10.1016/j.thorsurg.2011.09.003

DIAGNOSIS

The finding of specialized columnar epithelium, characterized by the presence of intestinal metaplasia (goblet cells), is the basis for the definition of Barrett esophagus proposed by the American College of Gastroenterology (**Fig. 1**).[8,9] Cytologically, goblet cells are barrel-shaped and have a distended, mucin-filled cytoplasm. Histochemically, goblet cells contain acid mucins that stain positively with alcian blue at pH 2.5.[11] In addition, columnar cells between goblet cells may resemble either gastric foveolar cells (incomplete intestinal metaplasia) or intestinal absorptive cells (complete intestinal metaplasia).[12] Unlike normal gastric foveolar cells, which contain neutral mucin, nongoblet columnar cells in Barrett esophagus often contain alcian blue–positive acid mucin, although the intensity of staining is not as great as that seen in goblet cells (**Fig. 2**).[13] In the absence of goblet cells, however, a diagnosis of Barrett esophagus should not be rendered based solely on the presence of alcian-blue positivity in nongoblet columnar cells (columnar blues).

Criteria for the histopathologic diagnosis of dysplasia in Barrett esophagus require evaluation of (1) surface maturation, (2) glandular architecture, (3) nuclear cytology, and (4) associated inflammation and erosion/ulcers.[14–16] In the progression from no dysplasia to high-grade dysplasia, there are progressively more severe changes in the first 3 elements. In high-grade dysplasia, (1) surface maturation is lacking, (2) there is glandular crowding, often with marked

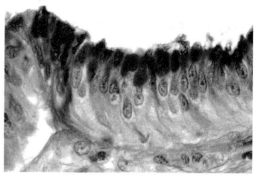

Fig. 2. Specialized columnar epithelium nongoblet columnar cells (columnar blues). In this alcian blue–stained section, presence of acidic mucin is detectable by its bright blue color. Cells that contain the acidic mucin, however, do not have the barrel-shaped morphology of goblet cells. Currently, the presence of these cells does not meet criteria for a diagnosis of Barrett esophagus.

distortion; (3) nuclei are hyperchromatic and nuclear membranes are irregular; and (4) inflammation may be minimal; however, it can be present, making the diagnosis more difficult (**Fig. 3**). High-grade dysplasia is characterized by markedly hyperchromatic cells extending onto the surface epithelium and complex glandular architecture with loss of nuclear polarity. Paradoxically, goblet cells diagnostic of intestinal metaplasia may be absent in dysplastic epithelium, presumably because they are overrun by the dysplastic epithelium.

Conceptually, differentiating of high-grade dysplasia from intramucosal cancer should be easy simply by examining the basement membrane. Intramucosal cancer occurs when neoplastic cells penetrate the basement membrane and infiltrate into the lamina propria or

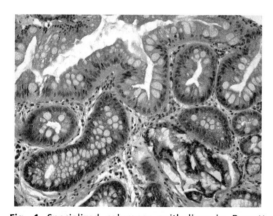

Fig. 1. Specialized columnar epithelium in Barrett esophagus. Currently, the histologic component of the diagnosis of Barrett esophagus requires the presence of intestinal metaplasia, as defined by the presence of goblet cells. Goblet cells have a characteristic shape because their cytoplasm is distended by acidic mucin, displacing the nucleus toward the bottom of the cell. In some hematoxylin-eosin stains, goblet cells may have a bluish hue.

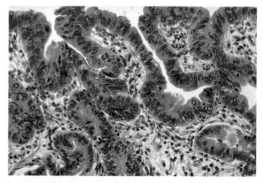

Fig. 3. High-grade dysplasia. There is glandular crowding with marked distortion and little intervening lamina propria. Nuclei are hyperchromatic and nuclear membranes are irregular. Inflammation is minimal and goblet cells are absent.

muscularis mucosae, but not below. Unfortunately, the basement membrane is not an easily identifiable robust structure, and it is often not obvious when cells penetrate this structure. Intramucosal cancer should be suspected, however, when there is (1) glandular crowding with essentially no intervening stroma (back-to-back glandular pattern), (2) cribriform growth pattern of glands (gland-within-gland pattern), and (3) cellular debris within at least 3 dilated, dysplastic glands within a high-power field.[17] It may be difficult to reach a consensus diagnosis of intramucosal cancer if these are the only findings that accompany those of high-grade dysplasia.

A significant problem facing pathologists is the long-recognized intraobserver and interobserver variation in the diagnosis of Barrett esophagus–related dysplasia. Given the subtle gradation of changes from baseline no dysplasia to intramucosal cancer, it is not surprising that this variation exists. It has been found most striking at the low end of the histologic spectrum (ie, distinguishing Barrett esophagus without dysplasia from changes that are indefinite for dysplasia or low-grade dysplasia).[14] A more recent study using κ statistical analysis, which accounts for agreement that may occur by chance alone, confirmed a high degree of intraobserver and interobserver variation in the separation of these diagnoses, even among pathologists with a special interest in gastrointestinal pathology.[16] This is particularly true in the assessment of biopsy specimens. Interobserver agreement among 7 gastrointestinal subspecialty pathologists was moderate for high-grade dysplasia but only fair for high-grade dysplasia with marked distortion of glandular architecture and intramucosal cancer.[18] Staining for various biomarkers has not been helpful in distinguishing high-grade dysplasia from intramucosal cancer.

Currently, the histologic finding of dysplasia is the best predictor for the development of cancer in patients with Barrett esophagus. The controversies and difficulties (listed previously) emphasize the need to obtain multiple opinions on difficult cases, preferably from pathologists with experience in evaluating these challenging biopsy specimens. Therapeutic strategies based on the histologic separation of high-grade dysplasia from intramucosal cancer should be viewed with skepticism, given the great difficulty in the histologic separation of high-grade dysplasia from intramucosal cancer.

SURVEILLANCE

It is clear that high-grade dysplasia is the immediate precursor lesion to esophageal cancer,

because it is frequently seen in the mucosa adjacent to such lesions. High-grade dysplasia, however, is also a marker of cancer elsewhere in the esophagus; approximately 30% to 40% of esophagi resected for high-grade dysplasia harbor an unsuspected cancer.[19–24] Surveillance esophagoscopy and biopsy with a goal of identifying dysplasia has become the standard of care for identifying those patients with Barrett esophagus at the highest risk of developing cancer. The benefit of this practice, however, has not been conclusively proved. The evidence is based on multiple reports demonstrating that patients with esophageal cancer who were undergoing surveillance had better survival than cancer patients not undergoing surveillance.[25–32]

The Seattle protocol of 4-quadrant biopsies using jumbo forceps taken every 1 cm of Barrett esophagus, with additional biopsies of suspicious lesions, has become the standard of care in surveillance. Frequency of surveillance is dictated by the pathologic diagnosis: patients with no dysplasia should have repeat esophagoscopy and biopsy in 3 to 5 years, those with low-grade dysplasia in 6 to 12 months, and those with high-grade dysplasia in 3 months in the absence of therapy.[4]

Dysplasia can be diffusely distributed throughout a segment of Barrett esophagus. In some patients, however, dysplastic alterations are focal, sometimes limited to a small area in one of many biopsy specimens. Even when using a rigorous endoscopic sampling technique, small dysplastic foci can be left unsampled (sampling error). The need for thorough sampling is further emphasized by the fact that many cases of high-grade dysplasia or early cancer are not associated with a grossly recognizable lesion.[15,33] Advanced esophagoscopy technologies, such as autofluorescence, confocal laser endomicroscopy, diffuse reflectance and light scattering spectroscopy, optical coherence tomography, narrow-band imaging, and chemoendoscopy can assist but have not replaced high-definition white light video esophagoscopy with sampling biopsy protocols in the detection of high-grade dysplasia in Barrett esophagus.

Once a diagnosis of dysplasia is made, subsequent biopsies without dysplasia should not lull a physician or patient into a false sense of security given the enormous problem of sampling error.

NATURAL HISTORY

The natural history of high-grade dysplasia is controversial and poorly understood. In a prospective study of patients with unifocal high-grade dysplasia and long-term follow-up, 8 of 15 (53%) patients progressed to either cancer or multifocal high-grade dysplasia within a mean of 37 months' follow-up.[34] The investigators concluded that unifocal high-grade dysplasia has a high risk for progressing to multifocal high-grade dysplasia or cancer and discouraged an observational approach when this diagnosis is rendered.

A single-institution study of 79 patients with high-grade dysplasia complicating Barrett esophagus reports a different natural history of high-grade dysplasia.[35] Rigorous esophagoscopy and biopsy detected a suspected cancer within the first year after detection of high-grade dysplasia in 4 patients. Of the 75 patients with high-grade dysplasia without detectable cancer after 1 year of intensive searching, only 12 (16%) subsequently developed cancer during a mean surveillance period of 7.3 years. Eleven of these 12 patients who developed cancers were considered cured with surgical or ablation therapy. Unlike Weston and colleagues, these investigators concluded that high-grade dysplasia without detectable cancer follows a relatively benign course in the vast majority of patients. Interestingly the 1099 patients with Barrett esophagus in this study, 737 (67%) had low-grade dysplasia, a percentage that far exceeds that of any other previously published study. One experienced gastrointestinal pathologist interpreted all of the biopsy specimens over a 20-year period.

A recent meta-analysis attempted to determine the incidence of cancer development in patients with high-grade dysplasia.[36] Of 3843 articles identified in a MEDLINE search, 196 were potentially relevant; however, only 4 studies met the inclusion criteria (histologically confirmed Barrett esophagus with high-grade dysplasia, no index cancers, and no ablative or surgical therapy). The crude incidence was 55.7 cancers per 1000 patient-years of follow-up (5.6% per year). With corrections this was estimated to be 6.6% per year.

Even more difficult to assess is the possibility of regression of high-grade dysplasia. Sampling error at esophagoscopy and biopsy, observer variation in the histopathologic diagnosis, and prior therapy make this contention impossible to prove or disprove.

MANAGEMENT OPTIONS
Observation

Previously, the absence of any therapy for high-grade dysplasia except esophagectomy made continued observation a viable treatment option. The poorly understood natural history of high-grade dysplasia, difficulties with its diagnosis, and introduction of new endoscopic therapies, however, have eliminated observation as a reasonable management strategy. Perhaps new surveillance technologies or discovery of biomarkers that identify patients with high-grade dysplasia who are at greatest risk of developing cancer may allow the return of observation as a viable management option.

Endoscopic Therapy

Mucosal ablation
Multiple single-institution studies have been published concerning endoscopic mucosal ablation. Two large randomized studies are available, however, and are important references that illustrate the role of this treatment option.

Endoscopic photodynamic therapy using porfimer sodium plus omeprazole was compared with omeprazole alone in the treatment of high-grade dysplasia in 208 patients, 138 treated and 70 controls. At a mean follow-up of 2 years, high-grade dysplasia was eliminated in 77% of the treatment group and, surprisingly, in 39% of controls (P<.0001). Cancer developed in 13% of the treatment group and 28% of controls (P = .006). Although there were no deaths in the treatment group, 69% experienced mild photosensitivity, 32% vomiting, and 20% chest pain; 36% developed esophageal strictures.[37] In a peculiar 5-year follow-up article in which "treatment failures" were censored and no further photodynamic therapy was administered to the remaining 61 patients, the treatment group had half the likelihood of progressing to cancer (15% vs 29%; P = .03) and longer time to cancer progression (P = .004).[38] These results, difficulties in administering this toxic treatment, and introduction of new technologies have rendered photodynamic therapy of historical interest alone.

Endoscopic radiofrequency ablation was compared with sham therapy in a multi-institutional randomized study[39]; 127 patients with dysplasia complicating Barrett esophagus were randomized 2:1 to receive treatment or none. Sixty-three had high-grade dysplasia and 64 had low-grade dysplasia. At 12-month follow-up of patients with high-grade dysplasia, complete eradication of dysplasia occurred in 81% of the treatment group and, surprisingly, in 19% of the sham group (P<.001). Among all patients, complete eradication of all intestinal metaplasia occurred in 77.4% of the treatment group and 2.9% of controls. Progression of high-grade dysplasia to cancer was reported in 2.4% of the treatment group and 19% of controls.

The mean number of treatments was 3.5. Three adverse events occurred, one upper gastrointestinal bleed in a patient receiving antiplatelet therapy for concomitant cardiovascular disease and 2 hospital admissions for chest pain. Chest discomfort was reported in 23 treatment patients and no sham patients. Chest discomfort resolved by day 8 after treatment. Strictures were reported in 5 patients (6%) and required a mean of 2.6 dilation sessions. Predictors of complete eradication were younger age, shorter Barrett segment, lower body mass index, and shorter history of dysplasia. These are short-term data, and the longevity and durability of radiofrequency ablation remain to be determined. Despite this lack of long-term follow-up, radiofrequency ablation is becoming the preferred therapy for high-grade dysplasia.

Mucosal resection

No similar studies exist for endoscopic mucosal resection; however, the largest single-institution study provides insight into this treatment option.[40] A reflection of the evolution in therapy for high-grade dysplasia, the treatment philosophy changed during this 6-year experience. Initially, ablation of remaining Barrett esophagus was not done; however, in the last 3 years of the study, ablation of remaining non-neoplastic epithelium was added to mucosal resection in patients who agreed to it. The results of this report are optimistic because intent-to-treat analysis was not performed. Of the 486 patients undergoing mucosal resection, only 349 were included in the study, 61 with high-grade dysplasia and 288 with intramucosal cancer. The results of treatment of high-grade dysplasia are not reported separately. At a mean follow-up of 64 months, complete response (defined as microscopic negative resection margins [R0] and one normal follow-up examination) occurred in 96.6% of patients, and 3.7% required esophagectomy. Metachronous neoplastic lesions developed in 21.5%, and 85% of these patients were successfully managed with further endoscopic therapy. There were 56 deaths, none due to Barrett adenocarcinoma. The overall 5-year survival was 84% and recurrence-free survival 77%. Predictors of recurrence were piecemeal mucosal resection, long-segment Barrett esophagus, no ablative therapy of Barrett esophagus after complete response, time to complete response greater than 10 months, and multifocal neoplasia. In the management of high-grade dysplasia, as in this study, mucosal resection has evolved into an adjunct to endoscopic ablative therapy.

Esophagectomy

Esophagectomy, the most aggressive therapy for high-grade dysplasia, has not been subjected to randomized studies. Multiple retrospective single-institution experiences have been reported.[19–24] The largest study reports the 27-year experience of esophagectomy in 134 patients with clinically diagnosed high-grade dysplasia[24]; 93% had high-grade dysplasia arising in Barrett esophagus. Fifty-seven percent were found to have high-grade dysplasia at esophagectomy, 34% intramucosal cancer, and 6% submucosal cancer. Two percent of these patients had regional lymph node metastases. Hospital mortality was 0.7%, and 5-year, 10-year, and 15-year survival percentages were 94%, 82%, and 75%, respectively. Older age and poor lung function predicted worse survival. Survival of the study group was similar to that of a matched cohort. Surprisingly, development of second nonesophageal primary cancers was 6.1 times expected.

The morbidity of esophagectomy is not inconsequential. Quality of life after esophagectomy was worse than for controls for at least 9 months.[41] By 5 years postoperatively, however, quality-of-life scores for patients with high-grade dysplasia or intramucosal cancer equaled or exceeded those of a matched population in 7 of 8 domains.[42] Eighty percent of these patients reported eating a normal or near-normal diet. After esophagectomy for high-grade dysplasia, quality of life at long-term follow-up was similar to national norms[43]; however, 50% of these patients required anastomotic dilation.

Anastomosis of the stomach to the esophagus at esophagectomy creates an environment that may foster reflux and may be complicated by development of Barrett esophagus in the esophageal remnant. A time-trend analysis of 231 esophagectomy patients followed a median of 3.5 years after esophagectomy estimated intestinal metaplasia to be found in 4% at 5 years and 16% at 10 years postoperatively.[44] No patient developed high-grade dysplasia or cancer. No variable other than passage of time was predictive of developing Barrett esophagus. Antireflux medications and higher anastomosis (closer to the upper esophageal sphincter) were associated with fewer reflux changes.

Although eradication of high-grade dysplasia is more likely to be complete and durable with esophagectomy, morbidity of this procedure has relegated it to a secondary treatment modality.

SUMMARY

The finding of high-grade dysplasia in Barrett esophagus is both a marker for future development of cancer and for the existence of synchronous cancer. A significant problem in management, however, is the intraobserver and interobserver variation in the histopathologic diagnosis of high-grade dysplasia in Barrett esophagus. As well, the natural history of high-grade dysplasia in Barrett esophagus is poorly understood. Thus, treatment decisions have been problematic. Recognition of both the difficulty in distinguishing high-grade dysplasia from intramucosal cancer and the similar long-term treatment outcomes has led to identical management strategies for these entities. The ability to preserve the esophagus with endoscopic mucosal ablation or resection and reduce morbidity of treatment, despite less complete and durable eradication of high-grade dysplasia compared with esophagectomy, has made endoscopic treatment the mainstay of therapy for high-grade dysplasia. Esophagectomy is reserved for treatment failures and for high-grade dysplasia not amenable to less-aggressive therapies.

REFERENCES

1. Wang KK, Sampliner RE. Updated guidelines 2008 for the diagnosis, surveillance and therapy of Barrett's esophagus. Am J Gastroenterol 2008;103: 788–97.
2. Fernando HC, Murthy SC, Hofstetter W, et al. The Society of Thoracic Surgeons practice guideline series: guidelines for the management of Barrett's esophagus with high-grade dysplasia. Ann Thorac Surg 2009;87:1993–2002.
3. American Gastroenterological Association, Spechler SJ, Sharma P, Souza RF, et al. American Gastroenterological Association medical position statement on the management of Barrett's esophagus. Gastroenterology 2011;140:1084–91.
4. Spechler SJ, Sharma P, Souza RF, et al. American Gastroenterological Association technical review on the management of Barrett's esophagus. Gastroenterology 2011;140:e18–52.
5. Paull A, Trier JS, Dalton MD, et al. The histologic spectrum of Barrett's esophagus. N Engl J Med 1976;295:476–80.
6. Lee RG. Dysplasia in Barrett's esophagus: a clinicopathologic study of six patients. Am J Surg Pathol 1985;9:845–52.
7. Reid BJ, Blount PL, Rubin CE, et al. Predictors of progression to malignancy in Barrett's esophagus: endoscopic, histologic and flow cytometric follow-up of a cohort. Gastroenterology 1992;102: 1212–9.
8. Haggitt RC. Barrett's esophagus, dysplasia and adenocarcinoma. Hum Pathol 1994;25:982–93.
9. Sampliner RE. Practice guidelines on the diagnosis, surveillance and therapy of Barrett's esophagus. Am J Gastroenterol 1998;93:1028–31.
10. Bhat S, Coleman HG, Yousef F, et al. Risk of malignant progression in Barrett's esophagus patients: results from a large population-based study. J Natl Cancer Inst 2011;103:1–9.
11. Haggitt RC, Reid BJ, Rabinovitch PS, et al. Barrett's esophagus. Correlation between mucin histochemistry, flow cytometry, and histologic diagnosis for predicting increased cancer risk. Am J Pathol 1988;131:53–61.
12. Levine DS, Rubin CE, Reid BJ, et al. Specialized metaplastic columnar epithelium in Barrett's esophagus. A comparative transmission electron microscopic study. Lab Invest 1989;60:418–32.
13. Offner FA, Lewin KJ, Weinstein WM. Metaplastic columnar cells in Barrett's esophagus: a common and neglected cell type. Hum Pathol 1996;27:885–9.
14. Reid BJ, Haggitt RC, Rubin CE, et al. Observer variation in the diagnosis of dysplasia in Barrett's esophagus. Hum Pathol 1988;19:166–78.
15. Reid BJ, Weinstein WM, Lewin KJ, et al. Endoscopic biopsy can detect high-grade dysplasia or early adenocarcinoma in Barrett's esophagus without grossly recognizable neoplastic lesions. Gastroenterology 1988;94:81–90.
16. Montgomery E, Bronner MP, Goldblum JR, et al. Reproducibility of the diagnosis of dysplasia in Barrett esophagus: a reaffirmation. Hum Pathol 2001; 32:368–78.
17. Patil DT, Goldblum JR, Rybicki LA, et al. Prediction of adenocarcinoma in esophagectomy specimens based upon analysis of pre-resection biopsies of Barrett's esophagus with at least high-grade dysplasia: a comparison of two systems. Am J Surg Pathol, in press.
18. Downs-Kelly E, Mendelin JE, Bennett AE, et al. Poor interobserver agreement in the distinction of high-grade dysplasia and adenocarcinoma in pretreatment Barrett's esophagus biopsies. Am J Gastroenterol 2008;103:2333–40.
19. Fernando HC, Luketich JD, Buenaventura PO, et al. Outcomes of minimally invasive esophagectomy (MIE) for high-grade dysplasia of the esophagus. Eur J Cardiothorac Surg 2002;22:1–6.
20. Tseng EE, Wu TT, Yeo CJ, et al. Barrett's esophagus with high-grade dysplasia: surgical results and long-term outcome—an update. J Gastrointest Surg 2003;7:164–70.
21. Reed MF, Tollis G Jr, Edil BH, et al. Surgical treatment of high-grade dysplasia. Ann Thorac Surg 2005;79:1110–5.
22. Sujendran V, Sica G, Warren B, et al. Oesophagectomy remains the gold standard for treatment of high-grade dysplasia in Barrett oesophagus. Eur J Cardiothorac Surg 2005;28:763–6.

23. Williams VA, Watson TJ, Herbella FA, et al. Esophagectomy for high grade dysplasia is safe, curative and results in good alimentary outcome. J Gastrointest Surg 2007;11:1589–97.

24. Rice TW, Murthy SC, Mason DP, et al. Esophagectomy for clinical high-grade dysplasia. Eur J Cardiothorac Surg 2011;40:113–9.

25. Corley DA, Levin TR, Habel LA, et al. Surveillance and survival in Barrett's adenocarcinoma: a population based study. Gastroenterology 2002;122:633–40.

26. Cooper GS. Endoscopic screening and surveillance for Barrett esophagus: can claims data determine its effectiveness? Gastrointest Endosc 2003;57:914–5.

27. Streitz JM, Andrews CW, Ellis FH. Endoscopic surveillance of Barrett's esophagus: does it help? Thorac Cardiovasc Surg 1993;105:383–8.

28. Peters JH, Clark GW, Ireland AP, et al. Outcome of adenocarcinoma arising in Barrett's esophagus in endoscopically surveyed and nonsurveyed patients. J Thorac Cardiovasc Surg 1994;108:813–22.

29. van Sandick JW, van Lanschot JJB, Kuiken BW, et al. Impact of endoscopic biopsy surveillance of Barrett's esophagus on pathologic stage and clinical outcome of Barrett's carcinoma. Gut 1998;43:216–22.

30. Incarbone R, Bonavina L, Saino G, et al. Outcome of esophageal adenocarcinoma detected during endoscopic biopsy surveillance for Barrett's esophagus. Surg Endosc 2002;16:263–6.

31. Ferguson MK, Durkin A. Long-term survival after esophagectomy for Barrett's adenocarcinoma in endoscopically surveyed and nonsurveyed patients. J Gastrointest Surg 2002;6:29–35.

32. Fountoulakis A, Zafirellis K, Donlan K, et al. Effect of surveillance of Barrett's oesophagus on clinical outcome of oesophageal cancer. Br J Surg 2004; 91:997–1003.

33. Falk GW, Rice TW, Goldblum JR, et al. Jumbo biopsy forceps protocol still misses unsuspected cancer in Barrett's esophagus with high-grade dysplasia. Gastrointest Endosc 1999;49:170–6.

34. Weston AP, Sharma P, Topalovski M, et al. Long-term follow-up of Barrett's high-grade dysplasia. Am J Gastroenterol 2000;95:1888–93.

35. Schnell TG, Sontag SJ, Chejfec G, et al. A Long-term nonsurgical management of Barrett's esophagus with high-grade dysplasia. Gastroenterology 2001;120:1607–19.

36. Rastogi A, Puli S, El-Serag HB, et al. Incidence of esophageal adenocarcinoma in patients with Barrett's esophagus and high-grade dysplasia: a meta-analysis. Gastrointest Endosc 2008;67: 394–8.

37. Overholt BF, Lightdale CJ, Wang KK, et al, International Photodynamic Therapy Group for high grade dysplasia in Barrett's Esophagus. Photodynamic therapy with porfimer sodium for ablation of high-grade dysplasia in Barrett's esophagus: international partly blinded, randomized phase III trial. Gastrointest Endosc 2005;62:488–98.

38. Overholt BF, Wang KK, Burdick S, et al. Five-year efficacy and safety of photodynamic therapy with Photofrin in Barrett's high-grade dysplasia. Gastrointest Endosc 2007;66:460–8.

39. Shaheen NJ, Sharma P, Overholt BJ, et al. Radiofrequency ablation in Barrett's esophagus with dysplasia. N Engl J Med 2009;360:2277–88.

40. Pech O, Behrens A, May A, et al. Long-term results and risk factor analysis for recurrence after curative endoscopic therapy in 349 patients with high-grade intraepithelial neoplasia and mucosal adenocarcinoma in Barrett's oesophagus. Gut 2008;57:1200–6.

41. Blazeby JM, Farndon JR, Donovan J, et al. A prospective longitudinal study examining the quality of life of patients with esophageal carcinoma. Cancer 2000;88:1781–7.

42. Moraca RJ, Low DE. Outcomes and health-related quality of life after esophagectomy for high-grade dysplasia and intramucosal cancer. Arch Surg 2006;141:545–51.

43. Headrick JR, Nichols FC 3rd, Miller DL, et al. High-grade esophageal dysplasia: long-term survival and quality of life after esophagectomy. Ann Thorac Surg 2002;73:1697–702.

44. Rice TW, Goldblum JR, Rybicki LA, et al. Fate of the esophagogastric anastomosis. J Thorac Cardiovasc Surg 2011;141:875–80.

Evidence-Based Review of the Management of Cancers of the Gastroesophageal Junction

Chaitan K. Narsule, MD[a], Marissa M. Montgomery, BA[b], Hiran C. Fernando, MD, FRCS[a],*

KEYWORDS

- Esophageal cancer • Gastroesophageal junction cancer
- Cardia tumor • Esophageal adenocarcinoma
- Neoadjuvant chemotherapy
- Neoadjuvant chemoradiotherapy • Mucosal ablation

The management of esophageal cancer continues to be a challenging problem for surgeons and oncologists. Despite improvements in surgical outcomes and techniques, survival for patients with evidence of nodal involvement remains poor. For this reason, neoadjuvant chemotherapy, with or without radiation, is often used, although not in a consistent fashion. Several randomized trials have been performed, but the results are difficult to interpret because of differences in the methods of preoperative staging, inclusion and exclusion criteria used in those trials, and type of esophagectomy performed.

Results are generally better for patients with an early-stage cancer. However, increased use of endoscopic therapies that allow for preservation of the esophagus are being reported for these patients.

In this article, we review the currently available evidence supporting the use of neoadjuvant and adjuvant therapies for esophageal cancer. Additionally, we review the evidence supporting the role of endoscopic therapies for early-stage esophageal cancer. For this article, we performed a search of the PubMed database for English-language articles using the following terms: early-stage esophageal cancer, T2N0 esophageal cancer, neoadjuvant chemotherapy, neoadjuvant chemoradiotherapy, and definitive chemoradiation for esophageal cancer. From this search, we selected 46 articles for inclusion in this article. This included 12 randomized trials, of which 10 were multicenter studies. The randomized trials were limited to the studies evaluating the role of neoadjuvant therapy. Recommendations were graded as indicated in Appendix 1.

STAGE I ESOPHAGEAL CANCER

Class I Recommendations

- It is reasonable to use esophagectomy to treat intramucosal (T1aN0) cancers of the esophagus. *Level of Evidence: B*

[a] Department of Cardiothoracic Surgery, Boston University School of Medicine, 88 East Newton Street, Robinson B-402, Boston, MA 02118, USA
[b] Boston University School of Medicine, 88 East Newton Street, Robinson B-402, Boston, MA 02118, USA
* Corresponding author.
E-mail address: hiran.fernando@bmc.org

Thorac Surg Clin 22 (2012) 109–121
doi:10.1016/j.thorsurg.2011.09.001
1547-4127/12/$ – see front matter © 2012 Elsevier Inc. All rights reserved.

- Esophagectomy is the preferred treatment for submucosal (T1bN0) cancers. *Level of Evidence: B*

Class IIb Recommendations

- Endoscopic therapy for superficial esophageal cancer, limited to the mucosa, may be reasonable when performed in experienced centers and in patients who will agree to undergo long-term surveillance endoscopy. In addition, intramucosal cancers treated endoscopically should meet the following criteria: size of 2 cm or smaller, well-differentiated or moderately differentiated pathology, no lymphatic or vascular invasion, and lateral and deep margins free of cancer after endoscopic mucosal resection. *Level of Evidence: B*

Endoscopic therapies are becoming increasingly popular for patients with high-grade dysplasia and superficial esophageal cancers. In part, this is related to concerns about excessive morbidity and mortality as high as 10% after esophagectomy.[1] More recent studies, however, such as a report using the Society of Thoracic Surgeons database, demonstrated a mortality of only 2.7% from a total of 2,315 esophagectomies performed in 73 centers.[2]

Investigators from the Cleveland Clinic previously reported a series of 122 patients with superficial esophageal cancer who underwent esophagectomy.[3] In this series, operative mortality was 2.5%, and 1-year, 5-year, and 10-year survival rates were 89%, 77%, and 68%, respectively. Eight (7%) patients had N1 disease, which was significantly associated with poorer survival. A more recent study from the University of Pittsburgh included 100 patients with T1 esophageal cancers who underwent esophagectomy.[4] Within this series, there were 29 intramucosal (T1a) cancers and 71 submucosal (T1b) cancers. N1 disease was identified in 21 patients. This occurred in 2 (7%) of the T1a patients and 19 (27%) of the T1b cancers. There were no 30-day mortalities. The overall 5-year survival for the entire cohort was 62%. For patients with N0 disease, this was 70% and for patients with N1 disease, this was 35%. Multivariate analysis also demonstrated that long tumor length ($\geq$2 cm) was a significant predictor of poor disease-free survival.

With the increasing use of endoscopic therapies for high-grade dysplasia, an alternative approach for superficial adenocarcinoma has been to combine endoscopic mucosal resection (EMR) with mucosal ablation. This approach was reported in a Dutch study involving 33 patients.[5] Patients with Barrett's esophagus and neoplastic lesions smaller than 2 cm in diameter, without evidence of lymph node involvement or submucosal involvement on endoscopic ultrasound (EUS), underwent EMR. Patients found to have T1b tumors were referred for resection, and patients with T1a tumors underwent follow-up with mucosal ablation for any remaining Barrett's esophagus. Twenty-eight patients were entered into the follow-up protocol after EMR. At a median follow-up of 19 months, 5 out of 26 patients had a recurrence of high-grade dysplasia, which was treated with repeat EMR.

A few centers have also described the use of endoscopic submucosal dissection for esophageal cancer.[6] One report involved 24 patients treated over 5 years. In this study, a curative resection was defined as occurring when the lateral and vertical margins of the tumor were free of cancer, there was no submucosal invasion deeper than 500 μm from the muscularis mucosa, and lymphatic or vascular invasion was absent. Additionally, any poorly differentiated adenocarcinoma or tumor with signet-ring cells was considered to have a noncurative resection. Using these very strict criteria, 72% of patients had curative resections. At a median follow-up of 30.1 months, there was no local or distant recurrence.

Probably the largest reported experience of endoscopic therapy for superficial adenocarcinoma of the esophagus is that of the group from Wiesbaden, Germany.[7] This center previously reported a series of 144 resections in 100 patients. Each tumor was assessed according to the Japanese classification of early stomach cancers.[8] This classification is as follows: Type I (polypoid), Type IIa (flat and slightly elevated), Type IIb (flat and level), Type IIc (flat and depressed), and Type III (ulcerated). Patients with types I, IIa, IIb, and IIc tumors up to 20 mm were eligible for local therapy, which included EMR followed by mucosal ablation for the remaining non-neoplastic Barrett esophagus. Patients had to have an R0 resection, with one normal endoscopic examination to be considered a complete remission, before undergoing surveillance or mucosal ablation. Additionally, tumors with submucosal invasion or lymphatic or vascular invasion, and poorly differentiated tumors after EMR were not considered eligible for this protocol. At a mean follow-up of 36.7 months, recurrent or metachronous cancers occurred in 11% of patients. All were treated successfully with repeat EMR, with a calculated 5-year survival rate of 98%.

These studies suggest that an endoscopic approach may be reasonable for highly selected patients with superficial adenocarcinoma. However, it should be emphasized that these studies were performed in specialized centers where there was commitment, by patients and their treating physicians, to the rigorous long-term follow-up that is required to identify and treat any recurrent cancer that may occur. Additionally, the technique of endoscopic submucosal dissection described by the Japanese investigators[6] is challenging technically, and it is unlikely that this will be widely adopted. On the other hand, several centers are currently performing EMR, and as more data become available, endoscopic therapies may become the preferred treatment for low-risk intramucosal adenocarcinoma for appropriate patients.

CLINICAL T2N0M0 ESOPHAGEAL CANCER

Class IIb Recommendations

- It is reasonable to treat esophageal tumors that are clinically staged at T2N0M0 with either esophagectomy or with neoadjuvant therapy followed by esophagectomy. *Level of Evidence: B*
- Patients who are treated initially with esophagectomy and are found to have higher-stage cancers on pathology should be treated with adjuvant therapy. *Level of Evidence: B*

The literature concerning tumors clinically staged at T2N0M0 is limited. Because these patients clinically have no evidence of nodal disease, they are often treated with esophagectomy, as is similar to other early-stage, node-negative tumors.[9,10] Multimodality therapy for esophageal tumors, however, has become increasingly popular in response to poor outcomes after surgery alone for more advanced disease. Several of the larger randomized trials studying neoadjuvant therapy have included cT2N0M0 in their patient selection, but numbers are often small in this category and subset analyses for this patient group often have not been provided.[11–16] Given the inconclusive and controversial nature of this topic, it seems reasonable to examine whether patients staged at cT2N0M0 should receive neoadjuvant therapy or proceed directly to esophagectomy.

A major concern with cT2N0 disease is the accuracy of clinical staging. Overstaged patients may be subjected unnecessarily to neoadjuvant therapy and understaged patients may get inadequate therapy if proceeding directly to surgery. One study from the Cleveland Clinic found that the positive predictive value for esophageal carcinoma clinically staged at T2 was 23%.[17] The literature describes the percentage of overstaged

cT2N0M0 tumors as ranging from 54% to 66%,[17–21] with errors predominantly in tumor depth.[18] On the other hand, a large proportion of cT2N0 tumors are understaged, ranging from 20.1% to 55.0% in different series.[17–22] Staging errors in this category are unfortunately predominantly in nodal involvement,[18,22] a more significant adverse prognostic indicator than T stage. As such, cT2N0M0 cancers have a worse prognosis than pT2N0M0, simply by virtue of the large portion of understaged tumors.

On the basis of this large proportion of occult, node-positive cancers, many centers advocate induction therapy for cT2N0M0.[16,22,23] A retrospective study from the M. D. Anderson Cancer Center suggested that neoadjuvant therapy effectively downstages a significant number of patients, as their results demonstrated only 10% of patients with pathologic stage greater than T2N0M0,[23] in comparison with the expected percentage of 20.1% to 55.0% from the literature.[17–19,21,22] Although this may support the role of neoadjuvant therapy, this may also have significant negative implications for patients with overstaged tumors. Advocates of the surgery-first approach argue that tumors found to be node positive on pathology may be treated with adjuvant chemoradiation with good results, thereby sparing patients with overstaged cancers from unnecessary chemotherapy and radiation therapy.[18] Adjuvant therapy for node-positive disease, although common practice, is also a subject of debate as to actual effectiveness in prolonging survival.[18,24–28]

There are currently only 2 studies specifically addressing the management of cT2N0M0 esophageal cancer, both of which are single institution and retrospective in design. The first study, by Rice and colleagues,[18] was undertaken at the Cleveland Clinic, and the second was reported by Kountourakis and colleagues,[23] at the M. D. Anderson Cancer Center. In both studies, patients with cT2N0M0 were a relatively small proportion of their total esophageal cancer populations. Rice and colleagues[18] identified 61 patients with this stage over 18 years, and Kountourakis and colleagues[23] identified only 49 patients over 12 years, although the latter report was restricted to cT2N0M0 patients treated with neoadjuvant therapy followed by surgery.

The Cleveland Clinic study reviewed 61 patients with clinically staged T2N0M0 by computed tomography (CT) and endoscopic ultrasonography. Rice and colleagues[18] analyzed patients who had surgery alone (n = 45), surgery first followed by chemoradiation for pathologically more advanced disease (n = 8), and surgery preceded by induction chemoradiation therapy (n = 8).

Only 7 patients of the 53 who underwent surgery first were found to have pathologic T2N0M0 (13.2%); 17 patients (32.1%) were understaged and 29 patients (54.7%) were overstaged. Overall survival at 10 years for overstaged cT2N0M0 treated with surgery alone was approximately 50%, which was found to be similar to propensity-matched surgery-alone patients (non-cT2N0M0 patients with less than pT2N0M0). Overall survival for correctly staged pT2N0M0 was similar to patients with overstaged T2N0M0 treated with surgery alone. For clinically understaged patients, survival was poor unless followed by adjuvant therapy: 10% at 5 years versus 43% at 5 years ($P = .17$). The induction therapy group (n = 8) had poor outcomes; of the 7 deaths at 10 years, 5 were cancer related. Patients who had induction therapy also had a poorer 5-year survival compared with the other treatment strategies used, at 13% versus 52% ($P = .05$). From these results, the investigators concluded that cT2N0M0 esophageal cancers should be treated with surgery first, followed by adjuvant therapy if they are found to be of a pathologically higher stage; otherwise, surgery alone was sufficient. They did not recommend induction therapy for cT2N0M0, although they acknowledged the limitations of that recommendation because of the small number of patients treated with induction therapy in their study.

In the M. D. Anderson Cancer Center study, a retrospective review of 49 patients with cT2N0M0 esophageal carcinoma who were treated with neoadjuvant therapy followed by surgery was undertaken. Clinical staging was done by endoscopic ultrasonography as well as CT imaging. A mean overall survival of 92.6 months and 5-year survival of 64.1% was demonstrated at a median follow-up of 28.4 months (range, 1.60–141.07 months). Five patients (10%) had a pathologic stage higher than T2N0M0. Fifteen of 44 patients with adenocarcinoma, and 3 of 5 patients with squamous cell carcinoma ($P = .342$), had a pathologic complete response to induction therapy. Although this was a single-arm study, the overall survival is promising compared not only with the 51% survival for cT2N0M0 patients treated with surgery first in the Cleveland Clinic study but also compared with the 50% 5-year survival specifically for pT2N0M0 patients reported in another study by the Cleveland Clinic group.[29]

In summary, there is limited evidence supporting an "induction therapy first" strategy versus an "esophagectomy first" strategy for clinically staged T2N0M0 esophageal tumors. We believe there would be equipoise for a randomized study

of this patient group, but this may not be feasible because of the relative scarcity of cT2N0M0 tumors.

CLINICAL N1 OR T3N0 ESOPHAGEAL CANCER

Class I Recommendations

- It is reasonable to use neoadjuvant chemotherapy with or without radiation to treat locally advanced esophageal cancer, before esophagectomy. *Level of Evidence: A*

Class IIb Recommendations

- There is no evidence that the addition of radiation is superior to chemotherapy alone with respect to survival, when used as neoadjuvant therapy for esophageal cancer. *Level of Evidence: B*
- Definitive radiation and chemotherapy for locally advanced esophageal cancer is reasonable, but should reserved for the high-risk surgical patient, or patients with resectable disease who refuse resection. *Level of Evidence: B*

For this discussion, patients with locally advanced esophageal cancer are defined as those with resectable tumors that are clinically staged as T3N0 or any T stage with N1 disease.

Management of locally advanced esophageal cancer has traditionally been by surgical resection alone. However, survival is poor with patients often succumbing to metastatic disease. In an effort to improve the outcomes, many investigators have studied the use of both preoperative chemotherapy and preoperative chemoradiotherapy and its impact on overall survival, disease-free survival, and R0 resection rate. An issue when interpreting many of these reports is that they are not always restricted to locally advanced disease, staging is not uniformly undertaken, and the type of esophagectomy used also is not uniform.[11,12,30–37] Another issue is that each series may include both mid and lower esophageal tumors, requiring extrapolation of the results for gastroesophageal junction and cardia cancers specifically.

On the other hand, because of the relatively larger number of patients presenting with locally advanced esophageal cancer, and the poorer survival associated with these tumors, many of the reports are from multicenter phase III trials.

Neoadjuvant Chemotherapy Followed by Surgery for Locally Advanced Esophageal Cancer

In 1998, the North American Intergroup trial by Kelsen and colleagues[30] compared 213 patients who were randomized to undergo neoadjuvant chemotherapy with cisplatin and fluorouracil followed by surgery with 227 who were randomized to undergo surgery alone for esophageal adenocarcinoma or squamous cell carcinoma. Staging involved chest x-ray, barium esophagram, and CT of the chest and abdomen; importantly, endoscopic ultrasonography was not required. Eligible patients had resectable tumors defined as T1-3, any nodal stage, and M0. Adenocarcinoma was seen in 121 (53%) of 227 patients in the surgery group and 115 (54%) of 233 patients who received preoperative chemotherapy. Interestingly, although chemotherapy did not affect operative mortality, which was 6% for each arm, it did not significantly affect R0 resection rates either (62% of the preoperative chemotherapy group vs 59% in the surgery-only group). Moreover, although there were more patients with R1 resections in the surgery group compared with the preoperative chemotherapy group (15% vs 4%, $P = .001$), there was no difference in overall survival, median survival, or disease-free survival (**Tables 1** and **2**). Therefore, in this Intergroup trial, the use of preoperative chemotherapy did not lead to a survival benefit.

In a subsequent multicenter randomized trial[31] by the Medical Research Council in 2002, 400 patients randomized to treatment with neoadjuvant chemotherapy, consisting of cisplatin and fluorouracil followed by surgery, were compared with 402 patients randomized to undergo surgery alone for esophageal adenocarcinoma or squamous cell carcinoma. Patients with resectable disease of all stages were included. Ten percent of the tumors were in the cardia and 64% were in the lower third of the esophagus. Also, 9% of patients in both arms received preoperative radiotherapy at the direction of their clinician. As was the case in the Intergroup trial, the use of preoperative chemotherapy did not lead to an increase in operative mortality, which was 10% for each arm. However, there was a higher rate of R0 resection when preoperative chemotherapy was used (60% vs 54%, $P<.0001$), and this persisted even when patients who did not receive preoperative radiotherapy were considered separately (60% vs 53%, $P<.0001$). With a median follow-up of 36.9 months for the preoperative chemotherapy group and 37.9 months for the surgery group, a benefit was seen in terms of overall survival (at 2 years, 43% vs 34%, $P = .001$) and improved disease-free survival (see **Tables 1** and **2**) favoring the neoadjuvant group. Interestingly, this study was updated in 2009 in a report[32] with a median follow-up of 72 months that demonstrated an absolute 5-year survival of 23.0% for the neoadjuvant arm compared with 17.1% for the surgery arm ($P = .03$).

In 2006, the Medical Research Council Adjuvant Gastric Infusional Chemotherapy (MAGIC) trial[33] reported on 250 patients randomized to undergo neoadjuvant chemotherapy with 3 cycles of epirubicin, cisplatin, and fluorouracil followed by surgery and 3 more cycles of adjuvant chemotherapy (same regimen), and compared with 253 patients who underwent surgery alone for adenocarcinoma of the stomach, esophagogastric junction, or lower esophagus. Inclusion criteria required that patients have resectable disease that was stage II or higher, with a tumor of either the stomach or lower third of the esophagus. Staging was performed by chest radiography, CT imaging, endoscopic ultrasonography, or laparoscopy. Gastroesophageal junction tumors comprised only 28 (11.2%) of the cases in the perioperative chemotherapy arm and 30 (11.9%) cases in the surgery-alone arm. The use of perioperative chemotherapy did not affect the rate of perioperative complications (45.7% vs 45.3% for the surgery group) or 30-day operative mortality (5.6% vs 5.9% for the surgery group). Moreover, there was a survival benefit seen among the patients treated with perioperative chemotherapy (5-year survival of 36.3% vs 23%, $P = .009$) and there was a higher likelihood of progression-free survival (hazard ratio for progression, 0.66; 95% confidence interval 0.53 to 0.81, $P<.001$).

More recently, Ychou and colleagues[34] reported on 113 patients randomized to treatment with neoadjuvant chemotherapy of fluorouracil and cisplatin followed by surgery and compared with 111 patients treated with surgery alone for gastroesophageal adenocarcinoma. Patients included in the study had a histologically proven resectable tumor in the lower third of the esophagus, the gastroesophageal junction, or the stomach, and cases of in situ carcinoma were excluded from analysis. In this series, 144 (64%) patients had a gastroesophageal junction tumor. The use of preoperative chemotherapy did not affect perioperative morbidity (25.7% vs 19.1% for surgery-only group, $P = .24$) or operative mortality (4.6% vs 4.5% for the surgery group, $P = .76$), but it did improve the R0 resection rate (84% vs 74% in the surgery group, $P = .04$). In addition, the group treated with neoadjuvant chemotherapy had an improved overall survival (5-year rate of 38% vs 24%, $P = .02$) and disease-free survival (5-year rate of 34% vs 19%, $P = .003$).

In summary, preoperative chemotherapy seemed to improve overall and disease-free survival in 3 of the 4 trials described previously, although

Table 1
Prospective randomized trials of preoperative chemotherapy with overall survival

Author, Year	Cancer Stages Treated	Median Follow-Up	Groups	Patients Randomized	Operative Mortality	3-y Overall Survival	5-y Overall Survival	Median Survival, mo	P Value
Kelsen et al,[30] 1998	T1-3, Any N, M0	46.5 months	Neoadj	227	6%	23%	20%[a]	14.9	.53
			Surgery	213	6%	26%	23%[a]	16.1	
Medical Research Council,[31] 2002	NR	36.9 months	Neoadj	400	10%	33%[a]	22%[a]	16.8	.004
	No locally inoperable disease or mets	37.9 months	Surgery	402	10%	24%[a]	13%[a]	13.3	
MAGIC,[33] 2006	Stage II or higher	49 months	Neoadj	250	5.6%	45%[a]	36.3%	23[a]	.009
	No locally inoperable disease or mets		Surgery	253	5.9%	31%[a]	23%	20[a]	
Ychou et al,[34] 2011	No Stage 0	68.4 months	Neoadj	113	4.6%	NR	38%	NR	.02
			Surgery	111	4.5%	NR	24%	NR	

Abbreviations: MAGIC, Medical Research Council Adjuvant Gastric Infusional Chemotherapy trial; mets, metastasis; Neoadj, neoadjuvant chemotherapy; NR, not recorded in report.
[a] Data estimated from survival curves.

Table 2
Prospective randomized trials of preoperative chemotherapy with disease-free survival

Author, Year	Groups	3-y Disease-Free Survival	5-y Disease Free Survival	P Value
Kelsen et al,[30] 1998	Neoadj	18%[a]	16%[a]	.5
	Surgery	18%[a]	16%[a]	
MRC,[31] 2002	Neoadj	24%[a]	18%[a]	.0014
	Surgery	17%[a]	12%[a]	
MAGIC,[33] 2006	Neoadj	38%[a]	30%[a]	<.001
	Surgery	26%[a]	18%[a]	
Ychou et al,[34] 2011	Neoadj	NR	34%	.003
	Surgery	NR	19%	

Abbreviations: MAGIC, Medical Research Council Adjuvant Gastric Infusional Chemotherapy trial; MRC, Medical Research Council; Neoadj, neoadjuvant chemotherapy; NR, not recorded in report.
[a] Data estimated from survival curves.

stage-specific survival information was not provided. Also, the R0 resection rate was increased when preoperative chemotherapy was used in 2 trials. Neoadjuvant chemotherapy does not appear to affect operative mortality significantly.

NEOADJUVANT CHEMORADIATION FOLLOWED BY SURGERY FOR LOCALLY ADVANCED ESOPHAGEAL CANCER

Many centers favor the inclusion of radiation therapy as part of their neoadjuvant therapy for esophageal cancer. It is believed that the addition of radiation allows a higher complete response rate (which may translate into better survival) and higher R0 resection rates. On the other hand, concerns remain about increased morbidity with the inclusion of radiation. The following describes 6 recent prospective randomized trials addressing the efficacy of preoperative chemoradiation followed by surgery for esophageal carcinoma.

In 1996, Walsh and colleagues[12] reported on a single-center prospective trial that studied 58 patients randomized to treatment with multimodality therapy (specifically fluorouracil, cisplatin, and 40 Gy of radiation followed by surgery) and compared with 55 patients who underwent surgery alone for esophageal adenocarcinoma. For the series, 51.0% of the patients had a tumor of the lower third of the esophagus and 34.5% had a tumor of the cardia. In the multimodality group, 5 patients died (1 of whom died preoperatively

owing to hemorrhage from the tumor bed) compared with 2 patients in the surgery-alone group. At the time of surgery, there were more patients with positive nodes in the surgery-alone group than in the multimodality group (82% vs 42%, P<.001). The median follow-up for all patients was 10 months (range, 0.1–59.0 months). The median survival for the multimodality group was longer than for the surgery-alone group (16 vs 11 months, P = .01), and the 3-year survival rate was higher for the multimodality group compared with the surgery-alone group (32% vs 6%, P = .01). One concern with this study is that the 3-year survival in the surgery-only group was significantly lower than other studies using surgery alone. Additionally, staging was not uniformly undertaken even with the use of a CT scan, which was used selectively in patients with equivocal findings on chest radiographs or liver ultrasonograms.

In the following year, Bosset and colleagues[11] reported on a multicenter trial in which 143 patients were randomized to preoperative chemoradiation (consisting of cisplatin and 18.5 Gy) followed by surgery and were compared with 139 patients who underwent surgery alone for squamous cell carcinoma of the esophagus. Endoscopic ultrasonography was not used, and staging was based on chest CT imaging. The following stages were included: T1N0, T1N1, T2N0, T2N1, and T3N0. Tumors staged as T3N0 comprised 29.5% of the surgery group and 32.9% of the multimodality group. The use of multimodality therapy was not associated with a higher rate of perioperative complications (45% vs 36% for the surgery group, P = .249), but was associated with a higher operative mortality rate (12.3% vs 3.6% for the surgery group, P = .012). At a median follow-up of 55.2 months, there was no significant difference in overall survival, with a median survival of 18.6 months observed for both treatment groups. The group treated with preoperative chemoradiation, however, had a longer disease-free survival (estimated 3-year disease-free survival of 40% for the multimodality group vs 28% for the surgery group, P = .003, and 5-year disease-free survival of 32% vs 24%, P = .003).

Thereafter, in 2001, the University of Michigan group reported a study of 50 patients randomized to treatment with preoperative chemoradiation (cisplatin, vinblastine, fluorouracil, and 45 Gy of radiation) followed by transhiatal esophagectomy, and compared with 50 patients treated with surgery alone for either squamous cell carcinoma or adenocarcinoma of the esophagus.[38] Patients included in this study had tumors of the esophagus or gastroesophageal junction, and the staging process did not use endoscopic ultrasonography. Two patients (4%) died in the surgery arm, and 1 (2.1%) died in the multimodality group. After a median follow-up of 8.2 years, there was no significant difference in 3-year overall survival (30% for the multimodality group vs 16% for the surgery-alone group, $P = .15$) or disease-free survival (28% vs 16%, respectively, $P = .16$) between the groups.

Similarly, Burmeister and colleagues[35] reported on 128 patients randomized to treatment with neoadjuvant chemoradiation (cisplatin, fluorouracil, and 35 Gy of radiation) followed by surgery and compared with 128 patients treated with surgery alone for squamous cell carcinoma or adenocarcinoma of the esophagus. Eligible patients had to have resectable tumors of the esophagus and gastric cardia (as long as the tumor was mainly in the lower esophagus), and included T1-3, N0-1 tumors. Also, as endoscopic ultrasonography was not widely available at the time of the study, its use in staging was not mandatory. Tumors of the lower third of the esophagus comprised 77% of the multimodality group and 81% of the surgery-alone group. Although an increased R0 resection rate was seen in the multimodality group (80% vs 59% for the surgery group, $P = .0002$), there was no significant difference in overall survival or progression-free survival (**Tables 3** and **4**) after a median length of follow-up of 65 months.

In 2008, the CALGB 9781 trial by Tepper and colleagues[36] reported on 30 patients randomized to treatment with neoadjuvant chemoradiation (cisplatin, fluorouracil, and 50.4 Gy of radiation) followed by surgery who were compared with 26 patients treated with surgery alone for squamous cell carcinoma or adenocarcinoma of the esophagus from 1997 to 2000. Eligible patients had either a thoracic esophageal cancer or a gastroesophageal junction tumor with less than 2-cm spread into the cardia, and stages included T1-3, N0-1, and M0. Staging by either EUS or thoracoscopy/laparoscopy was recommended. In all, 17 (56.7%) of 30 patients in the multimodality arm and 20 (77%) of 26 patients in the surgery arm had a clinical stage of T3N0, 75% of all patients had adenocarcinoma, and only 25% had N1 disease. There was only one perioperative mortality, occurring in the surgery arm. This multicenter randomized trial closed early because of poor accrual. With a median follow-up of 6 years, the median survival was 4.48 years for the multimodality group compared with 1.79 years for the surgery-only group ($P = .002$), and 5-year survival was 39% for the multimodality group compared with 16% for the surgery only group ($P = .008$). Survival based on clinical stage was not reported. This study demonstrates a large and significant difference in

median survival favoring the use of neoadjuvant chemoradiation. However, there was an unusually high percentage (66%) of patients who were clinically staged as T3N0. Although this group of patients has a high probability of occult nodal disease, their behavior may be more favorable compared with patients with clinically positive nodal disease and may in part explain these results, which are superior to most other randomized trials.

More recently, Gaast and colleagues[37] of the CROSS study group presented the results of 175 patients randomized to treatment with preoperative chemoradiation (paclitaxel, carboplatin, and 41.4 Gy of radiation) followed by surgery and compared with 188 patients treated with surgery alone. Patients included in the study had either esophageal or gastroesophageal tumors, for clinical stages T2-3, N0-1. For all patients, 75.2% of the tumors were adenocarcinomas. There was no difference in the in-hospital mortality, which was 3.8% for the multimodality group and 3.7% for the surgery group. The R0 resection rate favored the multimodality group (92.3% vs 64.9% for the surgery group). With a median follow-up of 32 months, overall survival was significantly better (3-year survival 59% vs 48%, favoring the multimodality group, $P = .011$), and median survival was 49 months in the multimodality group and 26 months in the surgery group.

It is unclear whether there is an advantage of neoadjuvant chemoradiotherapy over neoadjuvant chemotherapy. Two randomized studies have attempted to address this.[39,40] The first study from Germany randomized patients with T3-T4NXM0 disease to chemotherapy (15 weeks) or induction chemotherapy (12 weeks) followed by chemoradiation (3 weeks) before surgery.[39] The study was designed to include 354 patients but closed because of poor accrual at 126 patients. There was no difference in R0 resection rates, but there was a higher complete pathologic response rate in the chemoradiation patients (15.6% vs 2.0%, $P = .03$). Perioperative mortality was higher after neoadjuvant chemoradiation compared with chemotherapy (10.0% vs 3.8%), but this difference was not statistically significant ($P = .26$). There was also a nonsignificant trend ($P = .07$) favoring 3-year survival after neoadjuvant chemoradiotherapy compared with surgery (47.7% vs 27.7%). The second study addressing this issue was an Australian randomized phase II study involving 75 patients.[40] Preoperative chemotherapy was used in 36 patients and preoperative chemoradiotherapy in 39 patients. There was no difference in toxicity. The histopathological complete response rate (31% vs 11%; $P = .01$) was significantly better in the chemoradiation

Table 3
Prospective randomized trials of preoperative chemoradiotherapy with overall survival

Author, Year	Cancer Stages Treated	Median Follow-Up	Groups	Patients Randomized	Operative Mortality	3-y Overall Survival	5-y Overall Survival	Median Survival, mo	P Value
Walsh et al,[12] 1996	NR	10 mo 8 mo	Multimodal Surgery	58 55	12% 4%	32% 6%	NR NR	16 11	.01
Bosset et al,[11] 1997	T1-3, N0-1	55.2 mo	Multimodal Surgery	143 139	12.3% 3.6%	36%[a] 34%[a]	26%[a] 24%[a]	18.6 18.6	.78
Urba et al,[38] 2001	NR. (Disease limited to esophagus/GEJ)	98.4 mo	Multimodal Surgery	50 50	4% 2%	30% 16%	20%[a] 10%[a]	16.9 17.6	.15
Burmeister et al,[35] 2005	T1-3, N0-1	65 mo	Multimodal Surgery	128 128	5% 5%	36%[a] 31%[a]	26% 24%	22.2 19.3	.57
Tepper et al,[36] 2008	T1-3, N0-1	72 mo	Multimodal Surgery	30 26	0% 4%	66%[a] 20%[a]	39% 16%	53.8 21.5	.002
Gaast et al,[37] 2010	T2-3, N0-1	32 mo	Multimodal Surgery	175 188	4% 4%	59% 48%	NR NR	49 26	.011

Abbreviations: GEJ, gastroesophageal junction; NR, not recorded in report.
[a] Data estimated from survival curves.

Table 4
Prospective randomized trials of preoperative chemoradiotherapy with disease-free survival

Author, Year	Groups	3-y Disease-Free Survival	5-y Disease-Free Survival	P Value
Walsh et al,[12] 1996	Multimodal	NR	NR	NR
	Surgery	NR	NR	
Bosset et al,[11] 1997	Multimodal	40%[a]	32%[a]	.003
	Surgery	28%[a]	24%[a]	
Urba et al,[38] 2001	Multimodal	28%	25%[a]	.16
	Surgery	16%	12%[a]	
Burmeister et al,[35] 2005	Multimodal	34%[a]	31%[a]	.32
	Surgery	26%[a]	24%[a]	
Tepper et al,[36] 2008	Multimodal	60%[a]	28%	.007
	Surgery	15%[a]	15%	
Gaast et al,[37] 2010	Multimodal	NR	NR	NR
	Surgery	NR	NR	

Abbreviation: NR, not recorded in report.
[a] Data estimated from survival curves.

group; however, there was no difference in the median overall and progression-free survivals.

In summary, these trials suggest a benefit with respect to overall survival with neoadjuvant chemotherapy and radiation for esophageal or gastroesophageal junction cancer compared with surgery alone. In addition, an increase in both the R0 resection rate and complete pathologic response rate occurs when preoperative radiation is included in the neoadjuvant protocol. The addition of radiation does not appear to improve survival rates, however, and may lead to increased toxicity compared with chemotherapy alone.

DEFINITIVE CHEMORADIATION FOR LOCALLY ADVANCED ESOPHAGEAL CANCER

A randomized study from France compared chemoradiation followed by resection to chemoradiation alone.[41] This study was limited to squamous cell carcinoma of the esophagus, and only included patients with T3N0-1 cancers. Randomization occurred after therapy was initiated, and evidence of a response to initial chemoradiation was seen. In their study of 444 patients, there was felt to be no benefit by the addition of surgery with similar 2-year survival rates (34% vs 40%, $P = .44$). There was more locoregional relapse ($P = .03$) and a greater need for esophageal stents (5% vs 32%, $P<.001$) in the patients receiving definitive chemoradiation. Another randomized study from Hong Kong compared esophagectomy with definitive chemoradiotherapy for mid and lower squamous esophageal cancers.[42] Salvage esophagectomy was allowed for patients with incomplete

response or recurrence. With this approach, the 80-patient study demonstrated no difference in overall or disease-free survival. A follow-up report, from the same study, demonstrated that surgery was associated with a short-term negative impact on quality of life seen at 6 months, which became insignificant by 2 years.[43] On the other hand, chemoradiation was associated with progressive deterioration in pulmonary function with longer follow-up.

The issue of toxicity after chemoradiation is even more relevant in older patients, as demonstrated in a recent retrospective study from the Massachusetts General Hospital.[44] In this study, involving 34 patients aged 75 years or older (median age 75.9 years), only 50% of patients were able to complete planned therapy. Grade 4 or higher toxicity occurred in 38.2% of patients, with 70.6% of patients requiring hospital admission. Overall survival at 2 years was 29.7%. It should be emphasized that the median Eastern Cooperative Oncology Group Performance Status was excellent, at 1 in this group of elderly patients before therapy.

In one recent retrospective analysis,[45] 266 patients had been treated with platinum-based chemotherapy and 50 Gy of radiotherapy. Fifty-three percent of the cancers were adenocarcinomas. Also, tumors of the lower third of the esophagus or the gastroesophageal junction comprised 56% and 5% of all patients, respectively. Additionally, 58% were T3 tumors, 25% were T4 tumors, and 11% had M1a disease. In this series, median survival was 20.6 months, and the 2-year, 3-year, and 5-year survival rates were 43.6%, 32.9%, and 19.5%, respectively.

Also, Hironaka and colleagues[46] compared 53 patients treated with chemoradiotherapy and 45 patients treated with surgery for T2-3, N-any, M0 squamous cell carcinoma of the esophagus in a retrospective report in 2003. Chemoradiotherapy consisted of 5-fluorouracil, cisplatin, and 60 Gy of radiation. Lower-third esophageal tumors comprised 51.0% of the tumors in the surgery group and 30.2% of the tumors in the chemoradiation group. Additionally, the chemoradiation group had more advanced stage tumors than the surgery group. A pathologic complete response was seen in 70% of the chemoradiotherapy group, and the R0 resection rate was 98% in the surgery group. The perioperative morbidity rate of the esophagectomy group, however, was very high at 64%, and included an anastomotic leak rate of 29%. There was a 4% operative mortality, and no chemoradiotherapy-related deaths. With a median follow-up period of 43 months in both groups, the 5-year survival rates for the chemoradiotherapy and surgery groups were not significantly different (46% vs 51%, respectively, $P = .47$). Locoregional recurrence rates were not addressed in this study.

Although most reports are from retrospective studies, it does appear that the survival after definitive chemoradiation from retrospective studies approaches that of surgery alone, leading some oncologists to advocate this approach particularly for patients with locally advanced cancer and comorbid disease that would increase the risk of resection. On the other hand, studies as described previously have demonstrated poorer local control and swallowing after definitive chemoradiation, and significant morbidity may occur in patients with good performance status who are elderly.[44] For this reason, the authors advocate a neoadjuvant approach, including resection for patients with T3N0-1 disease, but recommend esophagectomy alone for the elderly patient with a high performance status, because of better locoregional control and preservation of swallowing.

SUMMARY

The successful management of gastroesophageal cancers continues to be a challenge for gastroenterologists, surgeons, and oncologists. Paralleling outcomes in the management of other solid tumors, neoadjuvant therapy before surgical resection seems to offer an improved survival in advanced stages. Because of the rarity of this disease, mixed stages treated, variety of pathologies and locations, and types of surgical resections performed, identifying optimal treatment

strategies has been challenging. Given the unfortunate fact that this disease is on the rise, we will be able to add to the growing body of treatment strategies in the future, hopefully leading to improved results in the management of this complex and deadly disease.

REFERENCES

1. Bailey SH, Bull DA, Harpole DH, et al. Outcomes after esophagectomy: a ten year prospective cohort. Ann Thorac Surg 2003;75:217–22.
2. Wright CD, Kucharczuk JC, O'Brien SM, et al. Predictors of major morbidity and mortality after esophagectomy for esophageal cancer: A Society of Thoracic Surgeons General Thoracic Database Risk Adjustment Model. J Thorac Cardiovasc Surg 2009;137(3):587–95.
3. Rice W, Blackstone EH, Goldblum JR, et al. Superficial adenocarcinoma of the esophagus. J Thorac Cardiovasc Surg 2001;122:1077–90.
4. Pennathur A, Farkas A, Krasinskas AM, et al. Esophagectomy for T1 esophageal cancer: outcomes in 100 patients and implications for endoscopic therapy. Ann Thorac Surg 2009;87:1048–55.
5. Femke PP, Mohammed AK, Wilda D, et al. Endoscopic treatment of high-grade dysplasia and early stage cancer in Barrett's esophagus. Gastrointest Endosc 2005;61:506–14.
6. Yoshinaga S, Gotoda T, Kusano C, et al. Clinical impact of endoscopic submucosal dissection for superficial adenocarcinoma located at the esophagogastric junction. Gastrointest Endosc 2008;67:202–9.
7. Ell C, May A, Pech O, et al. Curative resection of early esophageal adenocarcinomas (Barrett's cancer). Gastrointest Endosc 2007;65:3–10.
8. Nishi M, Omori, Miwa K. Japanese Society for Gastric Cancer. Japanese classification of gastric carcinoma. 1st English edition. Tokyo: Kanehara; 1995.
9. Tougeron D, Richer JP, Silvain C. Management of esophageal adenocarcinoma. J Visc Surg 2011; 148(3):e161–70.
10. Mariette C, Piessen G, Triboulet JP. Therapeutic strategies in oesophageal carcinoma: role of surgery and other modalities. Lancet 2007;8:545–53.
11. Bossett JF, Gignoux M, Triboulet JP, et al. Chemoradiotherapy followed by surgery compared with surgery alone in squamous cell cancer of the esophagus. N Engl J Med 1997;337:161–7.
12. Walsh TN, Noonan N, Hollywood D, et al. A comparison of multimodal therapy and surgery for esophageal adenocarcinoma. N Engl J Med 1996;335:462–7.
13. Nygaard K, Hagen S, Hansen HS, et al. Pre-operative radiotherapy prolongs survival in operable

esophageal carcinoma: a randomized, multicenter study of pre-operative radiotherapy and chemotherapy—the second Scandinavian trial in esophageal cancer. World J Surg 1992;16:1104–9 [discussion: 1110].

14. Pennathur A, Luketich JD, Landreneau RJ, et al. Long-term results of a phase II trial of neoadjuvant chemotherapy followed by esophagectomy for locally advanced esophageal neoplasm. Ann Thorac Surg 2008;85:1930–6.

15. Le Prise E, Etienne PL, Meunier B, et al. A randomized study of chemotherapy, radiation therapy, and surgery versus surgery for localized squamous cell carcinoma of the esophagus. Cancer 1994;73:1779–84.

16. Schwer AL, Ballonoff A, McCammon R, et al. Survival effect of neoadjuvant radiotherapy before esophagectomy for patients with esophageal cancer: a surveillance, epidemiology, and end-results study. Int J Radiat Oncol Biol Phys 2008;72:449–55.

17. Rice TW, Blackstone EH, Adelstein DJ, et al. Role of clinically determined depth of tumor invasion in the treatment of esophageal carcinoma. J Thorac Cardiovasc Surg 2003;125:1091–102.

18. Rice TW, Mason DP, Murthy SC, et al. T2N0M0 esophageal cancer. J Thorac Cardiovasc Surg 2007;133:317–24.

19. Crabtree TD, Yacoub WN, Puri V, et al. Endoscopic ultrasound for early stage esophageal adenocarcinoma: implications for staging and survival. Ann Thorac Surg 2011;91(5):1509–16.

20. Shimpi RA, George J, Jowell P, et al. Staging of esophageal cancer by EUS: staging accuracy revisited. Gastrointest Endosc 2007;66:475–82.

21. Zuccaro G Jr, Rice TW, Vargo JJ, et al. Endoscopic ultrasound errors in esophageal cancer. Am J Gastroenterol 2005;100:601–6.

22. Stiles BM, Mirza F, Coppolino A, et al. Clinical T2–T3N0M0 esophageal cancer: the risk of node positive disease. Ann Thorac Surg 2011;92(2):491–6.

23. Kountourakis P, Correa AM, Hofstetter WL, et al. Combined modality therapy of cT2N0M0 esophageal cancer: the University of Texas M. D. Anderson Cancer Center experience. Cancer 2011;117:925–30.

24. Rice TW, Adelstein DJ, Chidel MA, et al. Benefit of postoperative adjuvant chemoradiotherapy in locoregionally advanced esophageal carcinoma. J Thorac Cardiovasc Surg 2003;126:1590–6.

25. Armanios M, Xu R, Forastiere AA, et al. Adjuvant chemotherapy for resected adenocarcinoma of the esophagus, gastro-esophageal junction, and cardia: phase II trial (E8296) of the Eastern Cooperative Oncology Group. J Clin Oncol 2004;22:4495–9.

26. Macdonald JS, Smalley SR, Benedetti J, et al. Chemoradiotherapy after surgery compared with surgery alone for adenocarcinoma of the stomach

or gastroesophageal junction. N Engl J Med 2001; 345:725–30.

27. Power DG, Reynolds JV. Localized adenocarcinoma of the esophagogastric junction—Is there a standard of care? Cancer Treat Rev 2010;36(5):400–9.

28. Xiao ZF, Yang ZY, Liang J, et al. Value of radiotherapy after radical surgery for esophageal carcinoma: a report of 495 patients. Ann Thorac Surg 2003;75:331–6.

29. Killinger WA, Rice TW, Adelstein DJ, et al. Stage II esophageal carcinoma: the significance of T and N. J Thorac Cardiovasc Surg 1996;111:935–40.

30. Kelsen DP, Ginsberg R, Pajak TF, et al. Chemotherapy followed by surgery compared with surgery alone for localized esophageal cancer. N Engl J Med 1998;339:1979–84.

31. Medical Research Council Oesophageal Cancer Working Party. Surgical resection with or without preoperative chemotherapy in oesophageal cancer: a randomised controlled trial. Lancet 2002;359: 1727–33.

32. Allum WH, Stenning SP, Bancewicz J, et al. Long-term results of a randomized trial of surgery with or without preoperative chemotherapy in esophageal cancer. J Clin Oncol 2009;27:5062–7.

33. Cunningham D, Allum WH, Stenning SP, et al. Perioperative chemotherapy versus surgery alone for resectable gastroesophageal cancer. N Engl J Med 2006;355:11–20.

34. Ychou M, Boige V, Pignon J, et al. Perioperative chemotherapy compared with surgery alone for resectable gastroesophageal adenocarcinoma: an FNCLCC and FFCD multicenter phase III trial. J Clin Oncol 2011;29:1715–21.

35. Burmeister BH, Smithers BM, Gebski V, et al. Surgery alone versus chemoradiotherapy followed by surgery for resectable cancer of the oesophagus: a randomised controlled phase III trial. Lancet Oncol 2005;6:659–68.

36. Tepper J, Krasna MJ, Niedzwiecki D, et al. Phase III trial of trimodality therapy with cisplatin, fluorouracil, radiotherapy, and surgery compared with surgery alone for esophageal cancer: CALGB 9781. J Clin Oncol 2008;26:1086–92.

37. Gaast AV, van Hagen P, Hulshof D, et al. Effect of preoperative concurrent chemoradiotherapy on survival of patients with resectable esophageal or esophagogastric junction cancer: results from a multicenter randomized phase III study [abstract 4004]. J Clin Oncol 2010;28(Suppl):15s.

38. Urba SG, Orringer MG, Turrisi A, et al. Randomized trial of preoperative chemoradiation versus surgery alone in patients with locoregional esophageal carcinoma. J Clin Oncol 2001;19:305–13.

39. Stahl M, Walz MK, Stushka M, et al. Phase III comparison of preoperative chemotherapy compared with chemoradiotherapy in patients with locally advanced

adenocarcinoma of the esophagogastric junction. J Clin Oncol 2009;27:851–6.

40. Burmeister BH, Thomas JM, Burmeister EA, et al. Is concurrent radiation therapy required in patients receiving preoperative chemotherapy for adenocarcinoma of the oesophagus? A randomized phase III trial. Eur J Cancer 2011;47:354–60.

41. Bedenne L, Michel P, Bouche O, et al. Chemoradiation followed by surgery compared with chemoradiation alone in squamous cancer of the esophagus: FFCD 9102. J Clin Oncol 2007;25(10): 1160–8.

42. Chiu PW, Chan AC, Leung SF, et al. Multicenter prospective randomized trial comparing standard esophagectomy with chemoradiotherapy for treatment of squamous esophageal cancer: early results from the Chinese University Research Group for Esophageal Cancer (CURE). J Gastrointest Surg 2005;9:794–802.

43. Teoh AY, Chiu PW, Wong TC, et al. Functional performance and quality of life in patients with squamous esophageal carcinoma receiving surgery or chemoradiation: results from a randomized trial. Ann Surg 2011;253:1–5.

44. Mak RH, Mamon HJ, Ryan DP, et al. Toxicity and outcomes after chemoradiation for esophageal cancer in patients age 75 or older. Dis Esophagus 2010;23:316–23.

45. Gwynne S, Hurt C, Evans M, et al. Definitive chemoradiation for oesophageal cancer: a standard of care in patients with non-metastatic oesophageal cancer. Clin Oncol 2011;23:182–8.

46. Hironaka S, Ohtsu A, Boku N, et al. Nonrandomized comparison between definitive chemotherapy and radical surgery in patients with T2-3NanyM0 squamous cell carcinoma of the esophagus. Int J Radiat Oncol Biol Phys 2003; 57(2):425–33.

APPENDIX 1

Classification of Recommendation

Class I: Conditions for which there is evidence and/or general agreement that a given procedure is useful and effective.

Class II: Conditions for which there is conflicting evidence or a divergence, or both, of opinion about the usefulness and efficacy of a procedure.

Class IIa: Weight of evidence favors usefulness and efficacy.

Class IIb: Usefulness and efficacy is less well established by evidence.

Class III: Conditions for which there is evidence or general agreement, or both, that the procedure is not useful and effective.

Level of Evidence

Level A: Data derived from multiple randomized clinical trials.

Level B: Data derived from a single randomized trial or from nonrandomized trials.

Level C: Consensus expert opinion.

Follow-up of Patients with Resected Thoracic Malignancies

Paul M. Claiborne[a], Clara S. Fowler, MSLS[b],
Ara A. Vaporciyan, MD[c],*

KEYWORDS

- Follow-up • Thoracic • Malignancy • Surgery • Guideline

The purpose of follow-up after resection of malignancy is twofold: (1) early detection of recurrence and new tumors to allow early intervention leading to improved outcome and (2) patient support and counseling. Following curative resection of thoracic malignances, depending on the type of cancer, patients will be considered high-risk for recurrence or development of second primaries. The efficacy of surveillance for early detection of malignancy coupled with the effectiveness of treatment directed at those malignancies will determine the need, type, and frequency of follow-up. Follow-up as a means of patient support and counseling is an effective tool to maintain the physician-patient relationship and implement a patient-centered approach to cancer care.

The authors review the relevant guidelines established by the American College of Chest Physicians (ACCP), the National Comprehensive Cancer Network (NCCN), the American College of Radiology (ACR), the Scottish Intercollegiate Guidelines Network (SIGN), the European Society for Medical Oncology (ESMO), and the National Institute of Health and Clinical Excellence (NICE), with the Royal College of Surgeons addressing the follow-up of resected thoracic malignancies. The authors also present pertinent previous and current studies that have shaped the evidence for follow-up in the major categories of thoracic malignancies as well as the limitations identified in the literature. The quality of the evidence for guideline recommendations generated by the originating group is included. The cost-effectiveness of follow-up is not directly addressed because high-level evidence is lacking and an accurate evaluation is beyond the scope of this work.

METHODS

The authors first identified 8 databases for the guidelines search, including National Guideline Clearinghouse, SIGN, American Society of Clinical Oncology (ASCO), NCCN, ACCP, National Health Service (NHS) Evidence, MEDLINE, and EMBASE. The authors then performed an extensive literature search in each database using a combination of keywords: follow up, surgery, surgical, surgeon, resected, lung cancer, non small cell lung cancer, NSCLC, small cell lung cancer, thymic carcinoma, thymoma, chest wall tumor, and mesothelioma.

For MEDLINE and EMBASE, the authors used the Ovid interface and the search strategy listed in **Table 1**.

The authors also searched PubMed using the keywords previously listed for pertinent literature to any guidelines not indexed in the other databases. This hand-searched list was reviewed and inclusion was based on the relevance to the topic, clear recommendations generated by the investigators, and the quality of the evidence

The authors have nothing to disclose.

[a] The University of Texas Medical School at Houston, 6431 Fannin, Houston, TX 77030-1503, USA

[b] Information Services, Research Medical Library, The University of Texas MD Anderson Cancer Center, 1515 Holcombe Boulevard, Box 1499, Houston, TX 77030, USA

[c] Department of Thoracic and Cardiovascular Surgery, University of Texas MD Anderson Cancer Center, 1515 Holcombe Boulevard, Box 1489, Houston, TX 77030, USA

* Corresponding author.

E-mail address: avaporci@mdanderson.org

Thorac Surg Clin 22 (2012) 123–131

doi:10.1016/j.thorsurg.2011.08.011

1547-4127/12/$ – see front matter Published by Elsevier Inc.

Table 1
MEDLINE and EMBASE search strategy

MEDLINE Search	Results	EMBASE Search	Results
(1) exp guideline/	20999	1. practice guideline/	181,441
(2) follow up.mp.	732916	2. follow up.mp.	832,173
(3) 1 and 2	857	3. 1 and 2	9434
(4) exp Thoracic Neoplasms/	190478	4. exp thorax tumor/	5175
(5) 3 and 4	27		
		5. lung cancer/or lung tumor/ or respiratory tract cancer/	123,081
		6. exp lung carcinoma	88704
		7. exp thymoma	11,123
		8. exp mesothelioma	9688
		9. 4 or 5 or 6 or 7 or 8	212,407
		10. 3 and 9	142

presented. The publications presented are intended to highlight findings noted in the guidelines presented by the various societies.

NON–SMALL CELL LUNG CANCER

In 2010, an estimated 222,520 cases of lung cancer will be diagnosed. Approximately 85% are non-small cell lung cancer (NSCLC) and 25% to 30% are diagnosed in stages 1 and 2.[1,2] Therefore, an estimated 47,000 to 57,000 patients will require surveillance annually. High-quality clinical guidelines that can recommend the most appropriate follow-up care are vital.

ACCP Guidelines

Methods
The ACCP published a guideline for the follow-up of patients with lung cancer in 2003 and have since updated this guideline in 2007 based on subsequent evidence. An evidence-based practice center, external to the ACCP, was identified to perform the literature search, with priority given to systematic reviews, meta-analysis, and current guidelines. The literature was reviewed and a writing committee was responsible for generating the recommendations.[3]

Recommendations were graded based on the quality of evidence and the balance of risks versus benefits (**Table 2**). Results were reviewed for consensus among the multidisciplinary review board.

Recommendations

1. Surgical follow-up should be performed for 3 to 6 months by the thoracic surgeon who performed the curative-intent procedure.[4] Special expertise is recommended for the postoperative course complicated by hospital readmission, loss of function, and chronic pain related to the procedure. After this time period, a tumor board should be convened and the clinician responsible for diagnosis should oversee the surveillance of the patient (**Table 2**). (2C)

Table 2
ACCP: relationship of strength of the supporting evidence to the balance of benefits to risks and burdens

Quality of Evidence	Balance of Benefits to Risks and Burdens			
	Benefits Outweigh Risks/Burdens	Risk/Burdens Outweigh Benefits	Evenly Balanced	Uncertain
High	1A	1A	2A	
Moderate	1B	1B	2B	
Low or very low	1C	1C	2C	2C

Reproduced from McCrory DC, Lewis SZ, Heitzer J, et al. Methodology for lung cancer evidence review and guideline development: ACCP evidence-based clinical practice guidelines (2nd edition). Chest 2007;132(Suppl 3):23S–8S; with permission. American College of Chest Physicians.

2. Surveillance for patients with resected NSCLC that have adequate pulmonary function and performance should be with a history and physical examination and either chest radiograph or computed tomography (CT) every 6 months for 2 years and then annually. Patients should be educated on symptoms of recurrence and advised to return immediately for evaluation (1C).
3. Surveillance should be with a multidisciplinary team. Oversight and coordination of care should be the responsibility of the diagnosing clinician (2C).
4. Blood tests, positron emission tomography (PET) scanning, sputum cytology, tumor markers, and fluorescent bronchoscopy have no proven benefit and are not recommended in asymptomatic patients (2C).
5. Smoking cessation should be strongly advised, with pharmacotherapy and counseling offered for those patients who are unable to quit smoking (1A).

These guidelines reviewed all curative intent therapy, including surgery, radiation, and chemotherapy. Recommendations are based on all curative treatments, not specifically surgical resection.

NCCN Guidelines

Methods
The NCCN uses a multicenter process for developing their guidelines, including the NCCN Guidelines Steering Committee, the NCCN Guidelines Panel, an institutional review, and a group of members that perform literature searches on the selected topic. The NCCN Guidelines Steering Committee, along with the panel chair, selects a group of expert clinicians to serve on the guidelines panel. The multidisciplinary guidelines panel develops new recommendations and guidelines using available literature, including meta-analysis and clinical trials. When high-level evidence does not exist, lower level evidence, such as case series, nonrandomized trials, and expert opinion, are used to develop their guidelines.[5] The recommendations are graded based on NCCN Categories of Evidence and Consensus (**Table 3**).

Recommendations

1. Surveillance for recurrence or new primary should be a history and physical examination every 4 to 6 months, with spiral contrast CT for 2 years and then annually with noncontrast CT. (2B)[6]

Table 3
NCCN categories of evidence and consensus

Category 1	Based on high-level evidence, uniform consensus that intervention is appropriate
Category 2A	Based on low-level evidence, uniform NCCN consensus that the intervention is appropriate
Category 2B	Based on low-level evidence, nonuniform NCCN consensus that the intervention is appropriate
Category 3	Based on any level of evidence, there is major NCCN disagreement that the intervention is appropriate

From the NCCN Clinical Practice Guidelines in Oncology (NCCN Guidelines(tm)) for [non–small cell lung cancer] V[3.2011](c) 2011 National Comprehensive Cancer Network, Inc. All rights reserved; with permission.

2. Smoking cessation with counseling and pharmacotherapy should be offered. (2A)
3. PET scanning and brain magnetic resonance imaging (MRI) are not indicated. (2A)

The NCCN did reference 2 studies, the National Lung Screening Trial (NLST, preliminary results) and the International Early Lung Cancer Action Program (I-ELCAP). I-ELCAP was a nonrandomized study to assess the use of CT for screening of high-risk individuals for lung cancer.[7] The investigators, although documenting disagreement among panel members and without the final results of the NLST (unavailable when their guidelines were established), thought it was reasonable to include these results for recommendations for the surveillance of patients with resected malignancies.[6]

NICE/SIGN Guidelines

NICE and SIGN collaborated by sharing and dividing the literature search burden in the development of their respective guidelines. Each organization then independently reviewed and developed their guidelines.

Methods
NICE methods were the identification of new topic or preexisting guidelines needing an update, determination by the National Collaborating Center of the parameters of the intended guidelines, and development of the guideline by a multidisciplinary group reviewing available literature.

Stakeholders and an independent panel of experts review the recommendations.[8]

SIGN methods include a systematic review of literature through various databases. Selected papers are then evaluated by at least 2 multidisciplinary development group members. The recommendations are presented at conference and online for peer review, an independent expert review is performed, and an editorial group review by the SIGN council is done before finalization.[9]

Recommendations

Both NICE and SIGN were not able to identify any high-quality evidence in the literature for follow-up; however, the investigators gave recommendations based on expert opinion for good clinical practice.

Relevant recommendations to patient follow-up published by NICE in 2011 are (1) offering a follow-up appointment 6 weeks after the curative treatment, with future follow-up appointments offered with the intent to not rely on patient initiative to schedule future follow-up and (2) protocol-based follow-up by a clinical nurse specialist for patients with a life expectancy greater than 3 months.[8] Other 2005 recommendations are that the (1) patients' general practitioner should be informed of the intended follow-up schedule; (2) smoking cessation should be encouraged; (3) a nurse-led follow-up should be given as an option; and (4) follow-up should be every 3 months for the first 2 years and every 6 months for up to 5 years after the curative-intent therapy, with a chest radiograph included in the follow-up evaluation.[10]

A 2005 publication by SIGN gives no specific guideline recommendations regarding surveillance strategies, techniques, or a timeline for follow-up. However, the investigators do recommend an initial surgeon-led follow-up, with a later follow-up in compliance with established local clinical practice. The follow-up should be in collaboration with patients, the general practitioner, and the curative-treatment physician. Follow-up should be practice and patient specific according to the availability of local resources with the use of clinical nurse specialists.[9]

ESMO Guidelines

ESMO is a European professional organization founded in 1975. They have been formulating clinical practice guidelines outlining standard of care since 1999.[11]

Methods

ESMO guidelines are formulated by a multistep process consisting of a literature search for the topic and the designation of subject editors who select authors, oversee review and editing by a multidisciplinary group, and approve the final manuscript. Contributions to the sarcoma and lung cancer guidelines were also made through ESMO-supported conferences and meetings.[11]

Recommendations

The current ESMO recommendations for follow-up of NSCLC after curative-intent therapy are (1) careful vigilance for postoperative treatment complications during the first 3 to 6 months, (2) physical examination and CT scan every 6 months for the first 2 years and then annually, (3) PET is not recommended for routine follow-up because of the lack of conclusive evidence for the earlier detection of recurrence, and (4) smoking cessation.[12]

Relevant Nonsociety Publications

Specific studies investigating any improvement in the outcome with screening after curative resection are rare. In 1995, Walsh and colleagues[13] retrospectively studied the survival benefit of the follow-up of resected NSCLC in 358 patients. Regular follow-up, which varied among treating surgeons, included a combination of (chest radiograph, physical examination, CT, and others) at varying time intervals. Overall, follow-up tests and visits led to different treatment strategies and survival benefits in less than 3% of the total patients, and disease-free survival was the best predictor of survival. Survival benefit was defined as alteration of treatment of recurrence detected in asymptomatic patients versus symptomatic detection of recurrence. However, most patients were symptomatic at recurrence and diagnosed at unscheduled visits. Walsh and colleagues gave recommendations for follow-up with a physician or nurse practitioner, including chest radiography every 6 months for the first year postoperatively and every year thereafter.[13] Also in 1995, Virgo and colleagues[14] retrospectively followed 182 patients after curative resection and divided patients according to frequency of outpatient visits and diagnostic tests into intense and routine follow-up groups. No significant difference was found in patient outcomes between the groups, although the intensely followed group had a greater length of average survival. In 1999, Younes and colleagues,[15] found no significant difference in disease-free interval between a strictly followed group (routine follow-up with physical examination, chest radiography, CT, and liver function tests at set intervals) and a symptomatic follow-up group (follow-up when symptoms occurred, with less than 3 visits to following physician in first 2 years after the operation). All of these studies were plagued by their retrospective design and small numbers but they agreed that prospective data was necessary to properly identify if follow-up of the resected patients offers survival advantage.

Unfortunately, the prospective data that is now available has been inconclusive with contradicting results. Westeel and colleagues[16] prospectively followed 192 patients after resection. Like Walsh and colleagues, they found a significant survival benefit to intensified follow-up in a small subset of the patient population. These patients developed asymptomatic, limited recurrence. Most asymptomatic recurrences were diagnosed with CT scan and bronchoscopy, not routine follow-up procedures, such as history, physical examination, or chest radiograph.[16] Subotic and colleagues[17] prospectively found that the detection of recurrence was not improved by intensive follow-up in 88 patients because 88% of recurrence was found after the investigation of symptoms, and the overall survival of patients with intensive follow-up (monthly phone contact with patients or families about medical condition and new symptoms concurrently with regular follow-up) "was not different from usually reported rates in the literature."[17]

The National Lung Screening Trial

One final publication is by the NLST. Although not specifically addressing follow-up, this study will likely impact many of the previously presented guidelines. Only NCCN guidelines mentioned its preliminary results. The NLST was a multicenter, randomized controlled trial evaluating the effectiveness of low-dose spiral CT for the screening of high-risk individuals for lung cancer.[18] This study was designed with the statistical power of 90% for detecting a 20% reduction in mortality of those screened by CT as opposed to chest radiography. The inclusion criteria required were 55 to 75 years of age, at least a 30 pack-year history of cigarette smoking, and no more than 15 years since smoking cessation. The final results in the recent publication demonstrated a 20% reduction in lung cancer mortality in the CT screened population.

It is relevant to follow-up because patients with a prior history of lung cancer have a higher risk of developing a recurrence or a new lung primary than many of the patients enrolled in this study. Therefore, it is likely that some of the following guidelines may be adjusted to reflect these recent findings. The reader is encouraged to look for updates that reflect inclusion of the NLST findings into current guidelines. It should also be noted that the investigators acknowledged the likely extrapolation of their findings to base guideline recommendations for other patient populations stating "the current NLST data alone are, in our opinion, insufficient to fully inform such important decisions."[18] Although the decrease in mortality elucidated in the NLST patient population is significant, data specific for surveillance of patients with resected malignancies should be investigated.

Although many guidelines have established clinically reasonable recommendations for patient follow-up, there is a paucity of high-level evidence for surveillance of resected patients. Many if not most cancer centers and practices follow their own internally established protocols for patient surveillance conforming to patients' propensity for excessive follow-up, physicians' penchant for many diagnostic imaging and tests, and protocols followed during training.[2] Development of high-quality, reliable evidence should be the focus for future investigations to institute stronger guidelines.

ESOPHAGEAL

There were 16,640 new cases of esophageal cancer reported in 2010, with a reported 14,500 deaths attributed to esophageal cancer. According to the 2010 data, from 1999 to 2005 (among all races), 23% of esophageal cancers were diagnosed at a localized stage.[1] With 23% of esophageal cancers diagnosed at a localized stage and potentially resectable, an approximate 3800 patients will constitute a group that may benefit from surveillance. Although squamous-cell carcinoma, more common internationally and in Asia, has a moderate platform of evidence, data specific to adenocarcinoma, more common in the United States, is lacking. Subsequently, there are a limited number of guidelines published addressing follow-up.

NCCN Guidelines

The NCCN has published guidelines for follow-up of curative intent therapy, not specific for surgical resection, for patients diagnosed with esophageal cancer. They recommend the following: (1) a history and physical examination every 3 to 6 months for 1 to 2 years and every 6 to 12 months for 3 to 5 years and then an annual follow-up; (2) serum chemistry, complete blood count (CBC), imaging, upper endoscopy, biopsy as clinically indicated; (3) dilation for anastomotic stenosis; and (4) confirmation of HER2-neu testing if there is nonsurgical metastatic disease at presentation. (2A).[19]

ESMO Guidelines

ESMO found that evidence for scheduled follow-up after treatment does not exist, except when future surgical resection after chemotherapy might be considered. Routine follow-up should focus on symptomatic recurrence, patient support, and recovery.[20]

Other Guidelines

In 2002, the Association of Upper Gastrointestinal Surgeons of Great Britain and Ireland, the British Society of Gastroenterology, and the British Association of Surgical Oncology jointly published esophageal cancer guidelines that address follow-up. They also emphasize that without reliable evidence for directing follow-up protocol, follow-up should be concentrated on patient support and internal evaluation of outcomes by the treatment team. They recommend that clinical nurse specialists should be integrated into and used to aid in the follow-up of patients. Their recommendations were based on expert opinion and clinical experience in the absence of adequate clinical literature.[21]

Because of the dearth of evidence supporting reliable follow-up protocols for adenocarcinoma, this is a promising area of investigation. Investigators, with access to a large database of esophageal adenocarcinoma cases, would be able to develop a fundamental evidence base to guide surveillance.

THYMOMA

Thymoma is the most common anterior mediastinal malignancy in adults. Contrast CT is the current choice for detection, preoperative staging, and identification of operative versus nonoperative disease.[22] Complete surgical resection is often the desired curative modality for treatment. Unfortunately, late recurrence has occurred between 5 to 10 years after curative resection. The slow, indolent nature of many of these tumors makes identification of the benefits of surveillance more challenging.

NCCN Guidelines

The NCCN has published guidelines for the follow-up of thymoma recurrence in curative-intent therapy patients. Their recommendations are limited to annual CT for 10 years. The NCCN does not recommend screening for other primaries, although patients with thymoma are at a higher risk of developing a second malignancy (2A).[23]

ESMO Guidelines

ESMO has published guidelines with follow-up recommendations that are nonspecific for thymic tumors and include all neuroendocrine tumors. Their recommendations include follow-up for at least 10 years, assessment of biochemical markers (those elevated at diagnosis) specific to the patients' tumor type every 3 to 6 months, and CT or MRI annually for the evaluation of recurrence.[24]

Relevant Nonsociety Publications

Some investigators have presented evidence considering alternative modalities for the surveillance of thymoma recurrence in resected patients. El-Bawab and colleagues[25] conducted a retrospective study comparing CT and fluorine-18 fluorodeoxyglucose PET (FDG-PET) for detection of recurrent thymomas in 37 patients that underwent surgical resection (with additional radiation or chemotherapy on a patient-specific basis). They found a sensitivity and specificity of CT for detection of recurrent disease of 71% and 85%, respectively, and sensitivity and specificity of FDG-PET of 82% and 95%, respectively. They suggest that these findings should prompt further prospective investigation of FDG-PET imaging for the recurrence of thymoma. Limitations of that study included retrospective modality, patient sample size, and length of follow-up.

Mineo and colleagues[26] conducted a retrospective analysis of prognostic factors for the recurrence of disease in 88 patients with resected thymoma. Disease recurrence after resected thymoma was found to correlate with Masaoka stage, World Health Organization classification, and cell cycle gene expression proteins (p53, p21 and p27). Of these, cell cycle protein p27 expression rates, in association with p53 and p21, were found to have the highest correlation with disease-free survival. Further evaluation of thymoma gene expression proteins to assess the ability to identify patient/tumor-specific strategies and surveillance methods for recurrence was recommended. Limitations to this study are the retrospective modality; duration of follow-up; and additional treatment modalities, specifically radiation therapy, in study patients.

Additional work is necessary to determine the role of PET and gene expression markers for surveillance. New, more reliable study designs with larger patient populations are needed to consider the implementation of alternative surveillance techniques.

CHEST WALL TUMORS

Primary chest wall tumors are rare and surgical resection is the preferred curative treatment modality. Radical resection with wide negative margins is a significant prognostic factor for disease-free survival.

NCCN Guidelines

The NCCN has published guidelines for follow-up after surgical resection of chondrosarcoma, osteosarcoma, soft-tissue sarcomas, and desmoids tumors of the chest wall. The surveillance recommendations for chondrosarcoma are divided by low grade and intracompartmental and high grade or clear cell or extracompartmental. After surgical resection in low-grade and intracompartmental lesions, the NCCN recommends a follow-up consisting of physical examination, chest radiograph and lesion radiograph every 6 to 12 months for 2 years and then annually as appropriate (2A).[27]

In high-grade, clear-cell, or extracompartmental lesions, the NCCN recommends more intense follow-up consisting of physical examination, primary site imaging (chest radiograph or cross-sectional study) as indicated, with chest imaging every 3 to 6 months for 5 years and then annually for at least 10 years. Functional capacity should also be assessed on each office visit during the follow-up period (2A).[27]

For osteosarcoma, surveillance will consist of physical examination, chest imaging, CBC, and any other laboratory tests that are indicated, imaging of the primary site with the same technique used for workup, and reassessment of functional capacity during every visit. Patients should be scheduled for these follow-up techniques every 3 months for the first 2 years following the operation, every 4 months for year 3, every 6 months for years 4 and 5, and then annually (2A). PET or bone scan imaging can be considered if appropriate (2B).[27]

For soft-tissue sarcomas, rehabilitation with occupational and physical therapy until maximal function is achieved, history and physical examination and chest radiography (CXR or CT) every 3 to 6 months for 2 to 3 years, then every 6 months for 2 years, and then annually are recommended. If the primary site of the tumor is easily assessed with physical examination, then subsequent imaging is not necessarily required. Consideration of postoperative baseline and periodic primary site imaging, based on locoregional recurrence risk factors, is recommended (MRI, CXR, or CT). The likelihood of recurrence after 10 years is small and patient-specific follow-up should be initiated. (2A).[28]

For desmoid tumors, rehabilitation with occupational and physical therapy until maximal function is achieved, history, and physical examination and chest radiography (CXR or CT) every 3 to 6 months for 2 to 3 years and then annually is recommended. (2A).[28]

ACR Guidelines

The ACR has published guidelines related to imaging and follow-up of musculoskeletal tumors. These guidelines are not specific to location, type, or treatment modality of the tumor. Their recommendations are classified into 7 variants based on low grade, high grade, surveillance for metastasis, and locorecurrence.[29] The recommendations are graded as follows: 1, 2, 3 means usually not appropriate; 4, 5, 6 means may be appropriate; and 7, 8, 9 means usually appropriate. Specific recommendation details and methods can be found on the ACR Web site, www.acr.org, under appropriateness criteria for the follow-up of malignant or aggressive musculoskeletal tumors.

MESOTHELIOMA

Malignant pleural mesothelioma (MPM) is a rare neoplasm with an incidence in the United States of approximately 2000 to 3000 cases yearly, and 58% of these cases are caused by asbestos exposure.[30,31] Incidence is trending down in the United States because of the regulations limiting asbestos exposure in the population, and within the next 50 years asbestos is likely not to be a factor in development of MPM.

The median survival time regardless of stage is between 9 and 17 months, emphasizing the lack of effective, curative treatment modalities.[30] Current evidence is also not clear on the choice between different surgical approaches. Pleurectomy/decortications have a reported local and distant recurrence rate of 64% to 72% and 10% to 36%, respectively. Extrapleural pneumonectomy has a more favorable local recurrence rate of 31% to 65% and a distant recurrence rate of 41% to 44%.[30]

ESMO Guidelines

ESMO has published guidelines for MPM and recommends follow-up with CT and clinical evaluation on a symptomatic basis.[32] Low incidence, low median overall survival, and the absence of a consensus curative surgical technique, supports the lack of evidence for follow-up after resection.

Currently, there is not a uniform consensus for screening or the detection of recurrence of MPM in high-risk or asbestos-exposed individuals.

However, a recently described serum marker, mesothelin-related peptide, may be predictive of disease recurrence after surgical resection.[33]

SUMMARY

Overall, current evidence emphasizes that the investigation of follow-up for resected thoracic malignancies is well behind and much less dynamic than the investigation into the diagnosis and treatment of these diseases. With the subsequent advancements in surgical treatment and other curative modalities, the ability to detect and intervene with curative therapy at earlier stages of the disease in a growing portion of the current patient population will certainly benefit from higher-quality evidence. Until consensus recommendations based on reliable literature can be constituted, the follow-up of patients with resected thoracic malignancies will be variable among treatment institutions and offer inconsistent benefits to surveillance patients.

REFERENCES

1. Jemal A, Siegel R, Xu J, et al. Cancer statistics, 2010. CA Cancer J Clin 2010;60(5):277–300.
2. Edelman MJ, Schuetz J. Follow-up of local (stage I and stage II) non-small-cell lung cancer after surgical resection. Curr Treat Options Oncol 2002; 3(1):67–73.
3. McCrory DC, Lewis SZ, Heitzer J, et al. Methodology for lung cancer evidence review and guideline development: ACCP evidence-based clinical practice guidelines (2nd edition). Chest 2007;132 (Suppl 3):23S–8S.
4. Rubins J, Unger M, Colice G. Follow-up and surveillance of the lung cancer patient following curative intent therapy: ACCP evidence-based clinical practice guideline (2nd edition). Chest 2007;132(Suppl 3): 355S–67S.
5. National Comprehensive Cancer Network. NCCN Guidelines and Derivative Information Products: User Guide. 2011. Available at: http://www.nccn. org/professionals/transparency.asp. Accessed July 29, 2011.
6. Ettinger DS, Akerley W, Borghaei H, et al. NCCN clinical practice guidelines in oncology (NCCN guidelines): non-small cell lung cancer 2011; Version 3. 2011. Available at: http://www.nccn.org/ professionals/physician_gls/pdf/nscl.pdf. Accessed March 28, 2011.
7. Henschke CI, McCauley DI, Yankelevitz DF, et al. Early lung cancer action project: a summary of the findings on baseline screening. Oncologist 2001; 6(2):147–52.
8. National Collaborating Centre for Cancer. The diagnosis and treatment of lung cancer (update of NICE clinical guideline 24). NICE Clinical Guideline; 2011. (CG121). p. 198. Available at: http://guidance.nice. org.uk/CG121. Accessed November 6, 2011.
9. Scottish Intercollegiate Guidelines Network. Management of patients with lung cancer: a national clinical guideline 2005(80):66. Available at: http:// www.sign.ac.uk/pdf/sign80.pdf. Accessed March 28, 2011.
10. National Collaborating Centre for Acute Care. The diagnosis and treatment of lung cancer. NICE Clinical Guideline; 2005. (CG024). p. 107. Available at: http:// www.rcseng.ac.uk/publications/docs/lung_cancer. html. Accessed June 16, 2011.
11. Pavlidis N, Hansen H, Stahel R. ESMO clinical practice guidelines: development, implementation and dissemination. Ann Oncol 2010;21(Suppl 5): v7–8.
12. Crino L, Weder W, van Meerbeeck J, et al. Early stage and locally advanced (non-metastatic) non-small-cell lung cancer: ESMO clinical practice guidelines for diagnosis, treatment and follow-up. Ann Oncol 2010;21(Suppl 5):v103–15.
13. Walsh GL, O'Connor M, Willis KM, et al. Is follow-up of lung cancer patients after resection medically indicated and cost-effective? Ann Thorac Surg 1995;60(6):1563–70.
14. Virgo KS, McKirgan LW, Caputo MC, et al. Post-treatment management options for patients with lung cancer. Ann Surg 1995;222(6):700–10.
15. Younes RN, Gross JL, Deheinzelin D. Follow-up in lung cancer: how often and for what purpose? Chest 1999;115(6):1494–9.
16. Westeel V, Choma D, Clement F, et al. Relevance of an intensive postoperative follow-up after surgery for non-small cell lung cancer. Ann Thorac Surg 2000; 70(4):1185–90.
17. Subotic D, Mandaric D, Radosavljevic G, et al. Relapse in resected lung cancer revisited: does intensified follow up really matter? A prospective study. World J Surg Oncol 2009;7:87.
18. The National Lung Screening Trial Team. Reduced lung-cancer mortality with low-dose computed tomographic screening. N Engl J Med 2011; 365(5):395–409.
19. Ajani JA, Barthei JS, Bentrem DJ, et al. NCCN clinical practice guidelines in oncology (NCCN guidelines): esophageal and esophagogastric junction cancers (excluding the proximal 5cm of the stomach) 2011;Version 1. 2011. Available at: http://www.nccn. org/professionals/physician_gls/pdf/esophageal. pdf. Accessed March 28, 2011.
20. Stahl M, Budach W, Meyer HJ, et al. Esophageal cancer: clinical practice guidelines for diagnosis, treatment and follow-up. Ann Oncol 2010; 21(Suppl 5):v46–9.

21. Allum WH, Griffin SM, Watson A, et al. Guidelines for the management of oesophageal and gastric cancer. Gut 2002;50(Suppl V):1–23.

22. Marom EM. Imaging thymoma. J Thorac Oncol 2010;5(10 Suppl 4):S296–303.

23. Ettinger DS, Akerley W, Borghael H, et al. NCCN clinical practice guidelines in oncology (NCCN guidelines): thymomas and thymic carcinomas 2011;Version 1. 2011. Available at: http://www.nccn.org/professionals/physician_gls/pdf/thymic.pdf. Accessed March 28, 2011.

24. Oberg K, Hellman P, Kwekkeboom D, et al. Neuroendocrine bronchial and thymic tumours: ESMO clinical practice guidelines for diagnosis, treatment and follow-up. Ann Oncol 2010;21(Suppl 5):v220–2.

25. El-Bawab HY, Abouzied MM, Rafay MA, et al. Clinical use of combined positron emission tomography and computed tomography in thymoma recurrence. Interact Cardiovasc Thorac Surg 2010;11(4):395–9.

26. Mineo TC, Ambrogi V, Mineo D, et al. Long-term disease-free survival in patients with radically resected thymomas: relevance of cell-cycle protein expression. Cancer 2005;104(10):2063–71.

27. Biermann JS, Adkins DR, Benjamin RS, et al. NCCN clinical practice guidelines in oncology (NCCN guidelines): bone cancer 2011; Version 1. 2011. Available at: http://www.nccn.org/professionals/physician_gls/pdf/bone.pdf. Accessed April 24, 2011.

28. Mehren MV, Benjamin RS, Bui MM, et al. NCCN clinical practice guidelines in oncology (NCCN Guidelines): soft tissue sarcoma. The National Comprehensive Cancer Network; 2011. Version 1. 2011. Available at: http://www.nccn.org/professionals/physician_gls/pdf/sarcoma.pdf. Accessed March 28, 2011.

29. Roberts C, Daffner R, Weissman B, et al. ACR appropriateness criteria follow-up of malignant or aggressive musculoskeletal tumors. Reston (VA): American College of Radiology (ACR); 2008.

30. Tsao AS, Wistuba I, Roth JA, et al. Malignant pleural mesothelioma. J Clin Oncol 2009;27(12):2081–90.

31. Price B, Ware A. Time trend of mesothelioma incidence in the United States and projection of future cases: an update based on SEER data for 1973 through 2005. Crit Rev Toxicol 2009;39(7):576–88.

32. Stahel RA, Weder W, Lievens Y, et al. Malignant pleural mesothelioma: ESMO clinical practice guidelines for diagnosis, treatment and follow-up. Ann Oncol 2010;21(Suppl 5):v126–8.

33. Robinson BW, Creaney J, Lake R, et al. Soluble mesothelin-related protein: a blood test for mesothelioma. Lung Cancer 2005;49(Suppl 1):5109–11.

Index

Note: Page numbers of article titles are in **boldface** type.

A

ABG analysis. *See* Arterial blood gas (ABG) analysis
Ablative therapies
  percutaneous
    for early-stage NSCLC in high-risk patients,
      60–62. *See also* Percutaneous ablative
      therapies, for early-stage NSCLC in
      high-risk patients
ACCP. *See* American College of Chest Physicians
  (ACCP)
ACR. *See* American College of Radiology (ACR)
AF. *See* Atrial fibrillation (AF)
Age
  as factor in lung resection candidates, 48
  as factor in sublobar resection for early-stage
    NSCLC in high-risk patients, 58
American College of Chest Physicians (ACCP)
  guidelines for follow-up of patients with resection
    for NSCLC, 124–125
American College of Radiology (ACR)
  guidelines for follow-up of patients with resection
    for chest wall tumors, 129–130
Amiodarone
  in AF prevention after general thoracic surgery,
    16–17
Antibiotic(s)
  in thoracic surgery, **35–45**. *See also* Thoracic
    surgery, perioperative antibiotics in
Anticoagulant(s)
  perioperative management of, **29–34**
    dabigatran, 32
    dipyridamole, 32
    heparin, 32
    thienopyridines, 30–32
    warfarin, 29–30
  postoperative use of, 32–33
Anticoagulation
  in AF management after general thoracic surgery,
    20–21
Arterial blood gas (ABG) analysis
  in lung resection candidates, 52
Aspirin
  postoperative use of, 33
Atrial fibrillation (AF)
  after general thoracic surgery, **13–23**
    adverse effects associated with, 13
    causes of, 13–14
    prevention of, 14–17

      amiodarone in, 16–17
      beta blockers in, 17
      calcium-channel blockers in, 15–16
      magnesium in, 17
      preoperative beta blockers in
        continuation of, 14–15
    risk factors for, 13–14
    treatment of, **17–21**
      anticoagulation in, 20–21
  prevalence of, 13

B

Barrett esophagus
  defined, 101
  with high-grade dysplasia, **101–107**
    definitions related to, 101
    diagnosis of, 102–103
    management of
      endoscopic therapy in, 104–105
      esophagectomy in, 105
      mucosal ablation in, 104–105
      mucosal resection in, 105
      observation in, 104
    natural history of, 103–104
    surveillance for, 103
Beta blockers
  in AF prevention after general thoracic surgery, 17
  before general thoracic surgery
    postoperative continuation of
      in AF prevention, 14–15
Bone
  of chest wall
    primary sarcomas of, 79–80
Brachytherapy
  in sublobar resection for early-stage NSCLC
    in high-risk patients, 58
Bupropion
  in smoking cessation, 7–8

C

Calcium-channel blockers
  in AF prevention after general thoracic surgery,
    15–16
Cancer(s)
  colorectal
    pulmonary metastases and
      histopathology of, 96

Thorac Surg Clin 22 (2012) 133–137
doi:10.1016/S1547-4127(11)00143-5
1547-4127/12/$ – see front matter © 2012 Elsevier Inc. All rights reserved.

Cancer(s) (*continued*)
   esophageal. *See* Esophageal cancer
   lung. *See* Lung cancer
   renal cell carcinoma
      pulmonary metastases and
         histopathology of, 96–97
Cardiopulmonary exercise testing
   in lung resection candidates, 51
Cardiovascular disease
   as risk factor in lung resection candidates, 48–49
Cartilage
   of chest wall
      primary sarcomas of, 79–80
CFRT. *See* Conventionally fractionated radiation
   therapy (CFRT)
Chemoradiation
   induction
      vs. induction chemotherapy
         for lung cancer, 72
Chemotherapy
   induction
      vs. induction chemoradiation
         for lung cancer, 72
Chest wall sarcomas, **77–81**
   clinical evaluation of, 77–78
   described, 77
   primary
      cartilage and bone, 79–80
      soft tissue, 78–79
      special considerations, 80
Chest wall tumors
   resected
      follow-up of patients with, 129
Clopidogrel
   postoperative use of, 33
Colorectal cancer
   pulmonary metastases and
      histopathology of, 96
Conventionally fractionated radiation therapy (CFRT)
   for early-stage NSCLC in high-risk patients, 58
Counseling
   in smoking cessation, 3–4

D

Dabigatran
   perioperative management of, 32
   postoperative use of, 33
Deep vein thrombosis (DVT), **25–26**
   risk factors for, 25
   risk stratification in, 25
Dipyridamole
   perioperative management of, 32
   postoperative use of, 33
Drug(s)
   in smoking cessation, 4, 6
DVT. *See* Deep vein thrombosis (DVT)

Dysplasia(s)
   defined, 101
   high-grade
      Barrett esophagus with, **101–107**. *See also*
         Barrett esophagus, with high-grade
         dysplasia

E

Embolism
   pulmonary
      acute, **25–26**. *See also* Pulmonary embolism,
         acute
Empyema
   perioperative antibiotics for, 43
Endobronchial ultrasonography
   in NSCLC staging, 71–72
Endoscopic therapy
   for Barrett esophagus with high-grade dysplasia,
      104–105
ESMO. *See* European Society for Medical Oncology
   (ESMO)
Esophageal cancer
   clinical N1 or T3N0
      management of
         evidence-based review of, 112–115
   clinical T2N0M0
      management of
         evidence-based review of, 111–112
   locally advanced
      management of
         evidence-based review of
            neoadjuvant chemoradiation followed
               by surgery, 115–118
   resection of
      follow-up of patients with, 127–128
   stage I
      management of
         evidence-based review of, 109–111
Esophageal surgery
   perioperative antibiotics in, 39–41
Esophagectomy
   for Barrett esophagus with high-grade
      dysplasia, 105
European Society for Medical Oncology (ESMO)
   guidelines for follow-up of patients with resection
      for esophageal cancer, 128
   guidelines for follow-up of patients with resection
      for mesothelioma, 129–130
   guidelines for follow-up of patients with resection
      for NSCLC, 126
   guidelines for follow-up of patients with resection
      for thymoma, 128

G

Gastroesophageal junction
   cancers of

management of
evidence-based review of, **109–121**. *See also specific cancers*
clinical N1 or T3N0 esophageal cancer, 112–115
clinical T2N0M0 esophageal cancer, 111–112
neoadjuvant chemoradiation followed by surgery for locally advanced esophageal cancer, 115–118
stage I esophageal cancer, 109–111

H

Heparin
perioperative management of, 32
postoperative use of, 33

I

Induction therapy
for lung cancer, **67–75**
endobronchial ultrasonography in, 71–72
induction chemoradiation *vs.* induction chemotherapy, 72
local control and complete response after neoadjuvant treatment, 72–73
mediastinal nodal disease ipsilateral to T is relative contraindication to surgical resection as primary treatment modality, 68
meta-analysis interpretation, 73
neoadjuvant treatment in converting nonresectable into resectable tumor, 68
PET in, 71–72
in reduction of exploratory thoracotomies, 71–72
for superior sulcus tumors, 71
T4 N0 could benefit from primary surgery but is relatively rare presentation of NSCLC, 68, 71
technical issues related to, 72
VATS in, 71–72
for thymic malignancies, **83–89**. *See also* Thymic malignancies, induction therapy for

L

Lung cancer
diagnosis
smoking cessation and, 2
induction therapy for, **67–75**. *See also* Induction therapy, for lung cancer
non–small cell
early-stage
in high-risk patients, **55–65**. *See also* Non–small cell lung cancer (NSCLC), early-stage, in high-risk patients
smoking and, 2

Lung resection
candidates for
long-term disability as perioperative risk in, 52
physiologic evaluation of, **47–54**
ABG analysis in, 52
age as factor in, 48
cardiopulmonary exercise testing in, 51
cardiovascular risk in, 48–49
described, 47–48
nutritional status in, 48
pulmonary function testing in, 49
6-minute walk test/shuttle-walk test in, 51–52
spirometry in, 49–50
stair climbing in, 51
tumor-related anatomic considerations in, 50–51
pulmonary rehabilitation in, 52
smoking cessation in, 52
perioperative antibiotics in, 36–39, 41
duration of, 38
efficacy of, 36–38
selection of agents, 38
surgeon experience in, 49
Lung transplantation
perioperative antibiotics in, 40–43

M

Magnesium
in AF prevention after general thoracic surgery, 17
Mesothelioma
resected
follow-up of patients with, 129–130
Mestastasectomy
pulmonary, **91–99**. *See also* Pulmonary metastasectomy
Mucosal ablation
for Barrett esophagus with high-grade dysplasia, 104–105
Mucosal resection
for Barrett esophagus with high-grade dysplasia, 105

N

National Comprehensive Cancer Network (NCCN)
guidelines for follow-up of patients with resection for chest wall tumors, 129
guidelines for follow-up of patients with resection for esophageal cancer, 127
guidelines for follow-up of patients with resection for NSCLC, 125
guidelines for follow-up of patients with resection for thymoma, 128
National Institute of Health and Clinical Excellence/Scottish Intercollegiate Guidelines Network (NICE/SIGN)

National (*continued*)
   guidelines for follow-up of patients with resection
      for NSCLC, 125–126
National Lung Screening Trial (NLST)
   on follow-up of patients with resection
      for NSCLC, 127
NCCN. *See* National Comprehensive Cancer
   Network (NCCN)
Neoadjuvant treatment
   for lung cancer
      local control and complete response after,
         72–73
      stage III NSCLC, 73
NICE/SIGN. *See* National Institute of Health and
   Clinical Excellence/Scottish Intercollegiate
   Guidelines Network (NICE/SIGN)
Nicotine replacement therapy (NRT)
   in smoking cessation, 5–7
      contraindications to, 7
      label warning related to, 7
Nonnicotine medications
   in smoking cessation, 7–8
Non–small cell lung cancer (NSCLC)
   early-stage
      in high-risk patients, **55–65**
         percutaneous ablative therapies for, 60–62
         radiation therapy for, 58–60
         sublobar resection for, 55–58
      mortality data, 55
   resection of
      follow-up of patients with, 124–127
         ACCP guidelines for, 124–125
         ESMO guidelines for, 126
         NCCN guidelines for, 125
         NICE/SIGN guidelines for, 125–126
         NLST on, 127
         relevant nonsociety publications guidelines
           for, 126–127
   stage III
      neoadjuvant treatment for, 73
NRT. *See* Nicotine replacement therapy (NRT)
NSCLC. *See* Non–small cell lung cancer (NSCLC)
Nutritional status
   as factor in lung resection candidates, 48

O

Osteosarcoma
   pulmonary metastases and
      histopathology of, 96

P

Percutaneous ablative therapies
   for early-stage NSCLC in high-risk patients, 60–62
      cancer-specific survival after, 62
      in local and regional control, 60
      toxicity of, 60, 62

Perioperative smoking cessation, **1–12**. *See also*
   Smoking cessation, perioperative
PET. *See* Positron emission tomography (PET)
Positron emission tomography (PET)
   in NSCLC staging, 71–72
Pulmonary embolism
   acute, **26–27**
      diagnosis of, 27
      risk stratification in, 26–27
      treatment of, 27
Pulmonary function testing
   in lung resection candidates, 49
Pulmonary metastasectomy, **91–99**
   described, 91–92
   lymph node status assessment in, 93–94
   radiographic imaging in, 92
   surgical approach
      considerations in, 94–95
      extent of resection in, 95–96
   tumor histopathologies, 96–97
Pulmonary rehabilitation
   in lung resection candidates, 52

R

Radiation therapy
   for early-stage NSCLC in high-risk patients, 58–60
      CFRT, 58
      SBRT, 58–60
      toxicity of, 60
Rehabilitation
   pulmonary
      in lung resection candidates, 52
Renal cell carcinoma
   pulmonary metastases and
      histopathology of, 96–97

S

Sarcomas
   chest wall, **77–81**. *See also* Chest wall sarcomas
   described, 77
   pathology of, 77
   primary soft tissue, 78–79
SBRT. *See* Stereotactic body radiation therapy
   (SBRT)
6-minute walk test/shuttle-walk test
   in lung resection candidates, 51–52
Smoking cessation
   benefits of, 2
   lung cancer diagnosis and, 2
   in lung resection candidates, 52
   perioperative, **1–12**
      interventions for, 3–9
         best practice recommendations, 9
         bupropion, 7–8
         combination therapy, 8–9

counseling, 3–4
nonnicotine medications, 7–8
NRT, 5–7
contraindications to, 7
label warning related to, 7
pharmacotherapy, 4, 6
varenicline, 8
relapse after, 9
preoperative, 2–3
Soft tissue
of chest wall
primary sarcomas of, 78–79
Spirometry
in lung resection candidates, 49–50
Stair climbing
in lung resection candidates, 51
Stereotactic body radiation therapy (SBRT)
for early-stage NSCLC in high-risk patients, 58–60
Sublobar resection
for early-stage NSCLC in high-risk patients, 55–58
adjuvant brachytherapy in, 58
age as factor in, 58
extent of resection, 56
tumor size in, 56–58
Superior sulcus tumors
induction therapy for, 71
Surgical site infection
defined, 35

T

Thienopyridines
perioperative management of, 30–32
Thoracic malignancies
resected
follow-up of patients with, **123–131**
chest wall tumors, 129
esophageal cancer, 127–128
mesothelioma, 129–130
methods for, 123–124
NSCLC, 124–127. See also Non–small cell
lung cancer (NSCLC), resection of,
follow-up of patients with
thymoma, 128
Thoracic surgery
general
AF after
prevention of, **13–23**. See also Atrial
fibrillation (AF), after general thoracic
surgery, prevention of
perioperative antibiotics in, **35–45**. See also
specific indications, e.g., Lung resection,
perioperative antibiotics in
for empyema, 43
in esophageal surgery, 39–40
history of, 35–36

in lung resection, 36–39
in lung transplantation, 40–43
practice patterns of, 36–43
Thoracotomy(ies)
exploratory
PET, VATS, and endobronchial
ultrasonography in, 71–72
Thromboembolism
risk factors for, 29–30
venous. See Venous thromboembolism (VTE)
Thrombosis
deep vein, **25–26**
Thymic malignancies
induction therapy for, **83–89**
discussion, 85–87
stage III or greater
induction therapy for, 83–85
Thymoma
resection of
follow-up of patients with, 128
Tobacco use
economic costs of, 1
healthcare costs related to, 1
mortality related to, 1–2
prevalence of, 1
Transplantation
lung
perioperative antibiotics in, 40–43

U

Ultrasonography
endobronchial
in NSCLC staging, 71–72

V

Varenicline
in smoking cessation, 8
VATS. See Video-assisted thoracoscopic surgery
(VATS)
Venous thromboembolism (VTE)
defined, 25
guidelines for, 25–26
prevention of
duration of, 26
risk factors for, 26
Video-assisted thoracoscopic surgery (VATS)
in NSCLC staging, 71–72
VTE. See Venous thromboembolism (VTE)

W

Warfarin
perioperative management of, 29–30
postoperative use of, 33